Conversations About Asthma

Conversations About Asthma

Lawrence M. Lichtenstein, MD, PhD

*Director, Professor of Medicine
Johns Hopkins Asthma & Allergy Center
Johns Hopkins Bayview Research Campus
Baltimore, Maryland*

Kathryn S. Brown

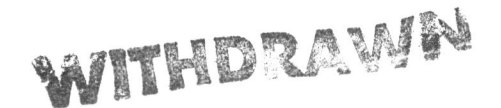

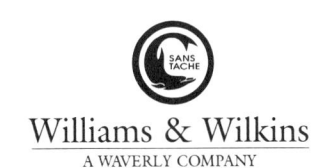

Williams & Wilkins
A WAVERLY COMPANY

BALTIMORE • PHILADELPHIA • LONDON • PARIS • BANGKOK
BUENOS AIRES • HONG KONG • MUNICH • SYDNEY • TOKYO • WROCLAW

Editor: David Charles Retford
Managing Editor: Jennifer Eckhoff
Developmental Editor: Kathleen H. Scogna
Production Coordinator: Marette D. Magargle-Smith
Project Editor: Robert D. Magee
Cover Designer: Graphic World, Inc.
Typesetter: Peirce Graphic Services, Inc.
Printer and Binder: Vicks Lithograph & Printing

Copyright © 1998 Williams & Wilkins

351 West Camden Street
Baltimore, Maryland 21201-2436 USA

Rose Tree Corporate Center
1400 North Providence Road
Building II, Suite 5025
Media, Pennsylvania 19063-2034 USA

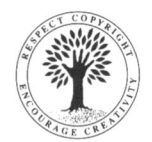

All rights reserved. This Book is protected by copyright. No part of this book may be reproduced in any form or by any means, including photocopying, or utilized by any information storage and retrieval system without written permission from the copyright owner.

Accurate indications, adverse reactions and dosage schedules for drugs are provided in this book, but it is possible that they may change. The reader is urged to review the package information data of the manufacturers of the medications mentioned.

Printed in the United States of America

First Edition

Library of Congress Cataloging-in-Publication Data

Lichtenstein, Lawrence.
    Conversations about asthma / Lawrence M. Lichtenstein, Kathryn S. Brown.
      p. cm.
    Includes index.
    ISBN 0-683-30434-8
    1. Asthma—Popular works.
RC591.L53 1997
616.2'38—dc21   97-26218
                                                                      CIP

The publishers have made every effort to trace the copyright holders for borrowed material. If they have inadvertently overlooked any, they will be pleased to make the necessary arrangements at the first opportunity.

To purchase additional copies of this book, call our customer service department at **(800) 638-0672** or fax orders to **(800) 447-8438**. For other book services, including chapter reprints and large quantity sales, ask for the Special Sales department.

Canadian customers should call **(800) 665-1148**, or fax **(800) 665-0103**. For all other calls originating outside of the United States, please call **(410) 528-4223** or fax us at **(410) 528-8550**.

Visit Williams & Wilkins on the Internet: **http://www.wwilkins.com** or contact our customer service department at **custserv@wwilkins.com**. Williams & Wilkins customer service representatives are available from 8:30 am to 6:00 pm, EST, Monday through Friday, for telephone access.

97 98 99 00
2 3 4 5 6 7 8 9 10

To Sam, whose Asthma will soon go away,
and to Jackson.

Preface

When I was a child, I struggled with asthma. It was the 1930s. At the time, doctors really didn't know much about asthma. When my parents took me to a physician, he suggested that our family spend every winter in Florida. It was common advice in those days. Sunny and warm, Florida seemed an ideal place for someone with asthma to stay healthy.

It wasn't.

For asthmatics, some of the most common irritants are dust mites, mold, and other substances you'll find in a wet climate, like Florida. While our doctor meant well, he didn't know enough about asthma to realize that I would wheeze and cough as much—if not more—during our winter vacations at the beach.

Things have changed a lot since then. Today, doctors understand that asthma attacks all begin with your environment. Certain "triggers," from allergens to pollutants to cold air, can aggravate your asthma. We also know that asthma is more than just an occasional outbreak of wheezing. It's a chronic disease that causes your airways to be slightly swollen, or inflamed, all the time. Along with this improved understanding, we have new drugs and better guidelines for treating asthma. In just the past few years, we've changed the way we approach the disease.

For you, the person with asthma, these advances are good news. Today, you can work with your doctor to control your asthma. Asthma is a very personal disease. That is, your symptoms and treatment may be different than anyone else's. That's why it's so important for you to get involved in managing your condition. It's not enough to simply take some medicine every once in a while. If you want to breathe more easily every day, you need to build a partnership with your health care provider and stay on top of your asthma. It's not hard—if you know how.

As I grew up, my asthma gradually improved. But I always remembered and wondered about the asthma attacks that affected my childhood. When I went to medical school, I quickly became interested in immunology, or the study of the immune system. Soon, I was researching the very symptoms that I knew so well. On a biological level, what leads to an asthma attack? On a practical level, what can you do about it? These kinds of questions have stuck with me throughout my career as a researcher and a doctor treating asthma patients. Today, I'm the director of the Asthma and Allergy Center at Johns Hopkins University in Baltimore. My colleagues and I are still asking asthma questions and finding answers to these questions.

This book will share the latest answers with you. As you read, you'll learn the basics of asthma and how to control it. I hope that, after reading this book, you'll feel a new confidence about your health. It's completely within your power to begin breathing more easily—and enjoying each breath a little more.

I'd like to extend a special thanks to Kathryn S. Brown and Delia K. Cabe for their assistance with this project.

Lawrence Lichtenstein. M.D., Ph.D.
Baltimore, Maryland

Contents

Preface

CHAPTER 1   Introduction: The Essentials of Asthma 1

CHAPTER 2   Working With Your Health Care Provider 11

CHAPTER 3   Asthma-Proofing Your World 21

CHAPTER 4   Asthma Medications 37

CHAPTER 5   Managing Your Asthma Day to Day 65

CHAPTER 6   Living With Asthma: Special Types of Asthma 79

CHAPTER 7   Living With Asthma: Pregnancy 89

CHAPTER 8   Living With Asthma: Everyday Situations 109

CHAPTER 9   Living With Asthma: Through The Years 123

CHAPTER 10   Frequently Asked Questions 139

CHAPTER 11   For More Information 145

Index 149

Chapter 1

Introduction: The Essentials of Asthma

A serious asthma attack is awful. It feels like you're sucking air through a straw, and it's all you can do to stay calm. But if you have asthma, you know that bouts of wheezing and coughing are only half the story. Asthma affects your life. In between asthma attacks, do you waste time worrying about the next one? Do these breathing battles make you feel frustrated? Have you ever missed out on something—from playing sports to taking a trip—because your asthma got in the way?

If you answered yes to any—or all—of these questions, this book is for you. Today, more than ever, you can control your asthma. New research, treatment guidelines, and drugs are all improving the way doctors approach asthma. Working with your health care provider, you can learn what triggers your asthma attacks and what medicine helps. What's more, you can create an "action plan" that keeps your asthma in check.

This book takes you beyond asthma's purely medical aspects. Today, one important trend in health care is to treat the whole person, not just the condition. This makes good health sense. After all, you don't just have asthma. You have a life. To feel confident about your health, you need to know how to fit asthma management into your life. You'll feel more in control when you do.

You'll also feel more in control if you get actively involved in managing your asthma from the very start. Talk to your doctor. When is your asthma worst? Does your medication help? You're the best person to answer these questions. Ask questions, too. Share your concerns with your health care provider. When you do, you'll learn a lot and feel better. Last, work hard to manage your asthma. You're the only person who can track your symptoms or take your medication every day.

Throughout this book, you'll learn all the things *you* can do to take control of your health.

You're not alone. Asthma affects at least 15 million Americans, a third of them children. And asthma is on the rise. Since 1980, asthma rates have more than doubled. We aren't sure, but we think the increase is due to a combination of better diagnosis; more outdoor pollution; and the trend toward tightly sealed homes and offices, in which dust mites, mold, and other indoor pollutants can build up.

As asthma's rate skyrockets, so does its impact. In a single year, asthma causes 2 million trips to the emergency room (ER) and 6 million visits to the doctor. It also causes 5,000 deaths, usually among people whose asthma has gone untreated. Asthmatic adults miss work; children miss school. And the cost is staggering. From ER and doctors' visits to medication, Americans spend $6 billion a year to ease their asthma symptoms.

TWITCHY LUNGS

What causes asthma? Asthma is a disease of the lungs, in particular, the bronchial tubes. The bronchial tubes, or "airways," carry air from your mouth to the air sacs in your lungs. If you have asthma, your lungs' airways overreact to things like allergens, cold air, or exercise. Doctors call this having "twitchy lungs." Sensing these stimuli, the inside lining of your airways begins to swell and make mucus. At the same time, the muscles outside your airways begin to tighten. This is the acute phase of asthma, or an asthma attack.

An asthma attack can last a few minutes, a few hours, or even a few days. Your asthma attacks may be mild, like an annoying cough, or severe, leaving you gasping for air. Most of the time, staying calm and taking your medication is the fastest way to end an asthma attack.

Unfortunately, asthma doesn't go away when your wheezing does. Even after an attack is over, asthma continues to inflame, or swell, the airways of your lungs. This is the chronic, inflammatory phase of asthma.

Over time, an army of cells—led by proteins called cytokines—can travel through your lungs, sometimes causing permanent damage to the tissue. When this happens, you can't breathe and use air as efficiently. Although you don't notice that your lungs are not working as well, these subtle changes make you vulnerable to more, and possibly more severe, asthma attacks in the future. That's why you need to take care of your asthma every day.

Asthma can be confusing because its symptoms and treatment differ so much from person to person. You might feel short of breath only at night, or you may be wheezy all day. Maybe your parents have asthma; maybe they don't. The drug that works so well for your best friend may do nothing for you. Everyone has their own asthma experience.

WHAT'S NEW IN ASTHMA TREATMENT TODAY?

Here's the good news: no matter what your experience, you can control your asthma. New drugs, better treatment guidelines, and ongoing medical research are changing the way doctors and their patients fight asthma. You, as a person with asthma, benefit.

In 1996, for example, the first entirely new class of asthma drugs in over 20 years began reaching pharmacy shelves. Called leukotriene antagonists, these oral medications ease asthma's inflammatory effects on a daily basis. In doing so, they help prevent asthma attacks and limit the long-term damage chronic asthma might do to your lungs.

A year later, the National Heart, Lung and Blood Institute (NHLBI), a government agency that funds and conducts medical research, released new treatment guidelines to help doctors better diagnose and manage asthma in all its varieties. Today, NHLBI urges health care providers to fight asthma more aggressively than in years past. That means diagnosing asthma in its early stages, trying powerful combinations of drugs, and carefully monitoring your progress as a patient. To manage asthma effectively, NHLBI suggests doctors and people with asthma follow four basic steps:

- Form a partnership with your doctor to explore and understand your asthma. What causes it? How severe is it? How does it respond to changes in your lifestyle, diet, and medication? Questions like these are best answered when you and your doctor work together.
- Control your environment to avoid asthma triggers.
- Find the right medications to stop your asthma attacks and treat your asthma on a daily basis.
- Use certain devices, like a peak-flow meter, to measure your breathing. It's difficult to assess your lung function based on just how you feel. Certain tests, however, can pick up changes in your breathing patterns before an asthma attack strikes.

From a research standpoint, our view of asthma is changing, too. In the past decade, scientists have begun to better understand and appreciate how asthma causes chronic lung inflammation, not just occasional attacks. At universities and drug companies across the country, researchers are studying the cells that cause your lungs to stay swollen and overreact. Some scientists are even hunting for genes that contribute to asthma. At the same time, researchers continue investigating the series of chemical reactions in the lungs that lead to an asthma attack. These efforts will lead to all-new asthma drugs in the future.

MAKING THE MOST OF THIS BOOK

This book draws upon these advances, as well as my own research and work with asthma patients over the last 35 years. In this book, you'll find the latest tips for controlling your asthma. You can read the book from beginning to end or use it as a reference guide, choosing just the chapters that discuss about your particular concerns. Be sure to share this book with family members so they can better understand your asthma, too.

The first half of this book explains the basics of asthma management and gives you the tools for self-care. The second half focuses on living with asthma and walks you through special asthma situations. Each chapter includes a summary and action plan to help you use what you learn.

At the end of the book, I'll discuss some questions frequently asked by my asthma patients. I've also included a chapter that lists government agencies, research organizations, and public health groups that offer asthma information or educational programs, many of which are free. Some organizations can suggest asthma support groups in your area. Because anyone with a chronic condition like asthma benefits from emotional support, I encourage you to contact these groups. You'll find strategies for coping with your asthma every day.

ASTHMA MANAGEMENT: ENVIRONMENT

The first step toward managing your asthma is a proper diagnosis. Depending on the severity of your asthma, you may work with a primary care provider, an allergist, or both. During the first visits, your doctor will take a medical history, do a physical examination, and test your lung capacity. These tools lay the groundwork for creating your personal asthma management plan. They're discussed at length in Chapter 2, "Working With Your Health Care Provider."

While your doctor is your partner, *you* have the most important job in managing your asthma. You can pay attention to and keep track of your asthma better than anyone else. Beginning an asthma management plan takes patience. You won't feel better in just a day or a week. But stick with it, and you will find yourself breathing more easily than you have in years. What's more, the quality of your life will improve.

After you are diagnosed with asthma, your first job is to notice your environment. Like most people with asthma, you probably realize you're unusually sensitive to some substances. When you are exposed to these so-called "triggers," your lungs overreact, and you get an asthma attack. Asthma triggers include allergens, or things that cause allergies, like dust mites, cockroach droppings, and animal hair; irritants in the air, like cigarette smoke; colds and other respiratory infections; exercise; and cold, dry air. The trick is to identify your personal triggers.

Allergens top the list of asthma triggers because allergies and asthma almost always go together. In both conditions, your body's immune system overreacts to its environment, causing inflammation. When you are asthmatic, that inflammation occurs in your lungs. For up to 90 percent of people with asthma, an allergic reaction launches asthma attacks. You can take certain steps to remove asthma-causing allergens from your life. Chapter 3, "Asthma-Proofing Your World," shows you how to uncover and eliminate the triggers that can bring on an asthma attack.

ASTHMA MANAGEMENT: MEDICATION

The next step toward controlling your asthma is medication. When I first started seeing patients more than 30 years ago, doctors only had a handful of drugs with which to battle asthma. Today, we have many drugs at our disposal. There are two basic types of asthma medicine. "Quick relievers," or bronchodilators, stop an asthma attack after it's begun. The second class of medication are anti-inflammatory drugs. These "long-term controllers" help prevent asthma attacks and protect your lungs on a daily basis.

Much like the triggers that spark your asthma, the medication that helps depends on your own condition. How often do you get asthma attacks? How bad are they? If you suffer mild asthma attacks once in a while, you may only need to take a quick reliever during those attacks. If, however, you get more serious or frequent asthma attacks, you probably need to take a long-term controller every day, too. Your health care provider will recommend the asthma medications you can try.

Asthma medications come in a variety of forms. Some are taken as pills, while others are inhaled. After evaluating your asthma, your doctor will choose the medication that's right for you. Inhaled medications can be tricky to use, so you need a doctor or nurse to show you the right technique—and probably more than once. The newest inhalers are getting simpler. Even so, some people, especially children, find it easier to inhale medicine using a machine called a nebulizer. Chapter 4, "Asthma Medications," explores the types of asthma drugs available and different ways to take them.

LIVING WITH ASTHMA

When you've got your asthma under control, you'll breathe better and feel better. Your next goal is simple: to stay this way. As you've learned, asthma doesn't just go away. Even with medication and a (mostly) trigger-free environment, an asthma attack is always possible.

Fortunately, you can prevent most attacks by monitoring your asthma. If you measure your breathing every day, you'll know when to take extra medicine or to carefully avoid asthma triggers. An easy-to-use device called a peak-flow meter can help you measure your lung function. You'll record your daily peak-flow measurements, as well as write down your asthma symptoms and medication in an asthma diary. In Chapter 5, "Managing Your Asthma Day to Day," you'll learn how peak-flow meters work and how to set up an asthma diary.

Also in Chapter 5, you'll learn how to react to the signs of a coming asthma attack. Most of the time, asthma doesn't strike suddenly. In as little as a few hours or as much as a couple of days before wheezing starts, your body warns you that something is wrong. These early signs are your call to action. Over the years, my patients have found that a nagging cough, itchy throat, or general feeling of fatigue means an asthma attack is on the way. Your health care provider can help you spot your personal asthma warning signs. Then, you can design an action plan for responding to these signs. The trick is to be ready.

Being ready isn't always easy, however. You may have a type of asthma that only occurs at certain times. In occupational asthma, for example, you only feel sick at work. You may be inhaling irritating substances like dust or vapors in carpeting, paint, and ventilation systems. What do you do? Chapter 6, "Living With Asthma: Special Types of Asthma" discusses how to manage these special types of asthma.

Also in Chapter 6, you'll find ways to manage your asthma off the job. One common type of asthma is exercise-induced. Some people stop playing sports because they get too wheezy and out of breath. But you don't have to sit on the sidelines. Olympic medal winners

Jackie Joyner-Kersee and Greg Louganis, for example, both have asthma. They—and hundreds of other athletes with asthma—prove that you can stay physically active. In this chapter, you can read up on the types of exercise and sports to try. You'll also learn how to get your airways ready, whether you're training for the Olympics or just enjoying the weekend.

No matter what type of asthma you have, changes in your general health can affect it. One important example is pregnancy. Asthma takes on new meaning if you're pregnant or hope to become pregnant. Suddenly, it's not just your disease anymore—it's a condition that can affect your unborn child. If untreated, your asthma may prevent your baby from getting enough oxygen in the womb. You could experience complications, too, ranging from high blood pressure to a complicated labor. About a third of the time, women discover their asthma gets worse during pregnancy.

The good news is that you can safely treat your asthma while pregnant. Your health care provider will help you find the right medications. Meanwhile, you can avoid the triggers that launch your attacks. Just as important, you and your doctor can monitor your baby's health during pregnancy, labor, and delivery. Moms-to-be who plan on breast-feeding can also learn whether asthma medication might affect their baby. "Chapter 7, Living with Asthma: Pregnancy" maps out the route to a healthy pregnancy for asthmatic moms and their babies.

Once you've addressed the big concerns about living with asthma, you may still need strategies for dealing with asthma in everyday life. Chapter 8, "Living With Asthma: Everyday Situations," addresses issues that may arise when you're feeling stressed; going on vacation; suffering frequent heartburn; having surgery; or getting sick with a cold, sinusitis, or another illness. In some cases, your asthma management may need to change.

So far we've discussed what asthma means to you and other adults. But what does it mean to children and their parents? Today, more than 1 in 20 children have asthma. For them, asthma can be scary, embarrassing, painful, or just plain annoying. If your child has asthma, you can help by learning about the disease and how it affects kids. The drugs, equipment, and even attitude toward asthma tends to be different. Pediatric asthma could take up a book by itself. Chapter 9, "Living with Asthma: Through the Years" covers some of the basics about asthma in children. This chapter also discusses asthma in the elderly. In older adults, asthma can be hard to distinguish from other respiratory conditions. Infections and certain types of medication may trigger asthma attacks. If you're an older adult, or if you have an elderly parent with asthma, your health care provider plays a more critical role than ever. Monitoring asthma requires regular check-ups at the doctor's office, and asthma medication may need to change fairly often.

Whether you're young or older, pregnant, athletic, working hard, or traveling, the message is the same: you can enjoy life without worrying that an attack of wheezing will sneak up on you.

SUMMARY: THE ESSENTIALS OF ASTHMA

- Asthma is a common disease that's on the rise. When you have asthma, your lungs overreact to certain things, like animal hair, dust mites, or cold air. Your airways start to swell, and you begin to cough, wheeze, or gasp for air.
- We do not have a cure for asthma, but we can treat it better than ever before.
- Asthma varies from person to person. Your asthma triggers, symptoms, and medication all depend on your own condition. Together, you and your doctor can create a personal asthma management plan that puts you in your control of your health.

ACTION PLAN

With your asthma under control, you can expect to live with far fewer asthma symptoms. You can exercise and play your favorite sports. You can sleep through the night. You can avoid missing school, work, or special family occasions. You also can avoid emergency room visits or hospital stays. You'll breathe better and feel better. Ready to get started? Here are the next steps you can take:

- Review the table of contents.
- Read Chapters 1–5. Find later chapters (Chapters 6–11) that address you particular concerns.
- Make a list of questions you'd like to ask your health care provider.
- Share the information in this book with family members or other loved ones.

Chapter 2

Working With Your Health Care Provider

Years ago, patients came in, listened to what their doctor had to say, and left. That has all changed. When it comes to your health, you should be an informed consumer, just as you are with other things in your life, like your car. You wouldn't take your car to a mechanic without asking lots of questions. First, you would go to a mechanic you could talk to and trust. You'd describe the problem. The mechanic would ask you questions to help him or her figure out what might be wrong. You'd find out what things needed repair. Afterward, you'd ask what to watch for—or do differently—to make your car run better. The same idea applies to your asthma care. This chapter is not just about going to the doctor. It's about building a partnership with your doctor.

The relationship between you and your health care provider is one of the most important aspects of managing your asthma. Your doctor is your ally and shares the same goal: improving your health. Together, you and your doctor will solve asthma-related problems and make sure that you stay healthy. This partnership takes commitment, time, and effort. But it's worth it. People with asthma who take an active role in their health care feel better, longer.

Whether you are already seeing a doctor for your asthma or are about to choose one, you need to know how to make the most of your office visits, from the first one on. During these appointments, you will:

- learn about asthma and self-management
- set treatment goals
- get encouragement and support
- tailor your asthma treatment plan

TALKING WITH YOUR DOCTOR

Before we discuss the specifics of your doctors' visits, let's go over what it means to be an informed health consumer. First, you need to learn about your asthma. Reading this book is a step in the right direction. You also might contact the resources listed in Chapter 11, "For More Information," to learn more.

When you're at the doctor's office, do more than just listen. Ask questions. Be honest about any concerns you might have. Honesty with your doctor is essential. You're not the only person who thinks asthma is complicated or confusing. Researchers have spent years trying to unravel the mysteries of this condition, and they're still hard at work on these efforts. Knowledge about asthma changes rapidly, so it's not surprising that you may have questions.

Your doctor has treated other people who have asthma and won't be surprised to hear your questions. Maybe you've heard that asthma medications are dangerous. They aren't—and your doctor can tell you why. Perhaps someone told you that asthma is all in your head. It's not. Your doctor—and this book—will show you that asthma is a real, treatable condition. Now's the time to ask questions and share any concerns you might have about your health. Below, I talk about ways to communicate with your doctor. I'll also share the kinds of questions to ask and information your doctor needs to know.

FINDING THE RIGHT DOCTOR

If you're looking for a doctor, think about what you want in a doctor. Do you prefer seeing a male or female doctor? Do you want the office to be near your workplace or close to home? Make a list and number the items from most to least important. Ask friends which health care providers they see and why they like—or don't like—them. Consider calling a doctor's office to find out more. If you belong to a health maintenance organization (HMO), call member services, and they can tell you whether a doctor is one of their providers. Some hospitals also maintain doctor referral services and can give you the phone numbers of doctors in your area. When you're speaking to someone in the doctor's office, feel free to ask questions like:

- Where has the doctor trained?
- Is the doctor board-certified in allergy?
- If the doctor has no specialty, does he or she have any particular areas of interest in asthma care?
- Is the doctor taking new patients?
- Does the doctor take my health insurance?
- What days/hours does the doctor see patients?
- How far in advance to I have to make appointments?
- In case of an emergency or urgent care visit (such as for an infection), how fast can I see the doctor?
- Who takes care of patients after hours or when the doctor is away?

When you make an appointment with a doctor, let the staff know the reason for your visit. For example, if you already know you have asthma but are having trouble with your symptoms, tell the receptionist. If it is your first visit, you may need a longer appointment so the doctor has time to learn your medical history. The first visit is a good time to begin building your relationship with your doctor. If you are seeing a doctor for the first time, be sure to have a copy of related medical records sent from your other doctor's office to the new one. The staff at your other doctor's office may ask you to sign a release form before they send your records.

SHOULD YOU SEE A SPECIALIST?

I believe that anyone diagnosed with asthma benefits from seeing an allergist. Your health plan may require you to get a referral from your primary care physician before you see an allergist or other specialist. Call your health plan to find out. If a referral is required, your primary care physician and you will decide together if you need to see an allergist.

An allergist is a physician who, after completing

medical school, did extra training to learn about allergies. An allergist can help you identify your asthma triggers, explain the subtleties of asthma, and put together a treatment plan that works for you. The National Asthma Education and Prevention Program Expert Panel Report II: Guidelines for the Diagnosis and Management of Asthma, issued in 1997, recommends that you see an allergist or pulmonologist (a lung specialist) if you have had a life-threatening asthma attack; have other conditions, such as sinusitis, severe rhinitis or gastroesophageal reflux disease (GERD) that complicate your asthma or its diagnosis; require additional testing, such as allergy skin testing or more lung function tests; have severe persistent asthma; or are considering allergy shots (immunotherapy).

After your asthma is under control, your primary care doctor can help you with routine asthma care. A primary care doctor is a physician who practices internal, general, or family medicine. He or she can treat most health problems and works with you to keep you healthy by following recommended asthma care guidelines given your age, sex, and medical history.

BEFORE GOING TO THE DOCTOR

During the time leading up to your appointment, start a list of things you want to discuss. Take notes. Write down questions and symptoms as soon as they occur to you. Plan to update your doctor about anything that has happened since your last visit. For example, you should let your health care provider know about a recent emergency room visit; a recent cold or other illness; any changes in your weight, sleep, energy level, or appetite; side effects from medication you may be taking; and any major stresses or changes in your life.

If you start an asthma diary (which you'll learn about in Chapter 5, "Managing Your Asthma Day to Day"), you might keep your "topics to discuss" list with that diary. This list will help jog your memory when you're at the doctor's office. On the day of your doctor's appointment, bring this list. Also bring your asthma diary and medications, including those prescribed by other health care providers and nonprescription drugs that you take regularly.

WHAT TO EXPECT DURING YOUR APPOINTMENT

You're finally at the doctor's office and thinking about what will happen during your appointment. Because you have done your homework, give yourself a pat on the back. You've come prepared and have some say in your visit. Don't forget that you and your health care provider are partners in your asthma care.

Your First Appointment

Asthma is sometimes hard to diagnose. Some people are not even aware that they have asthma. They might blame a cough on a lingering cold or the dry air outside. During your first visit, the goal is to determine whether it's asthma—or something else—that's making you wheeze and cough. Some conditions seem a lot like asthma. In children, an obstruction in the airways, such as one resulting from cystic fibrosis, can cause asthma-like symptoms. In adults, chronic bronchitis, emphysema, and congestive heart failure may all cause similar symptoms.

To make sure that you have asthma, your doctor will ask for your medical history, give you a physical examination, and perform certain tests. Your medical history will include questions like:

- What symptoms do you have?
- How often do you have symptoms? Every day? Less than once a week?
- In the last month, has coughing, wheezing, or shortness of breath bothered you at night? In the early morning? After running, moderate exercise, or other physical activity? During a particular season or time of year?
- Have you had colds that traveled into your chest or took more than 10 days to get over?

- What makes your symptoms occur or worsen? Better?
- Have you had a sudden severe episode or several episodes of coughing, wheezing, or shortness of breath?
- Have you tried any medications that help you breathe better? How often?
- Have you missed work or school because of your symptoms?
- How have your symptoms affected your lifestyle, activities, and family?

Your health care provider will also do a physical examination that focuses on your upper respiratory tract, chest and skin. During this examination, he or she will look to see if you have common signs of asthma, including hunched shoulders; sounds of wheezing (like whistling) during normal breathing; increased nasal secretions; swelling of the mucus membranes; or signs of allergic skin conditions, such as eczema.

What the doctor finds during the physical examination is somewhat subjective—findings can be interpreted differently by different doctors. So your health care provider will also need an objective test to diagnose your asthma. Depending on your history and the severity of your symptoms, your doctor may simply perform a spirometry test. A spirometer is an instrument that measures the air taken into and out of the lungs. Spirometry helps rule in asthma and rule out other causes. However, the results of this test are sometimes normal (between asthma attacks) in people with mild asthma. In that case, your doctor may give you a peak-flow meter—another device that measures lung function—to take home with you. Peak-flow meters come in various types, but they all do the same thing. The peak-flow readings will help you and your doctor make decisions about your treatment plan. You may also use the peak-flow meter throughout your treatment to monitor your asthma. I describe peak-flow meters and how to use one in Chapter 5, "Managing Your Asthma Day to Day."

Based on what you learn during this visit, your health care provider may think more tests are useful. Further tests might include a chest X-ray, allergy testing, and evaluation for gastroesophageal reflux disease (GERD). Whenever you need a medical test, feel free to ask your doctor:

- Why do I need this test?
- What will this test involve?
- Do I need to prepare for the test?
- Are there any complications from this test?
- What will the test tell us?
- When will the results come back? Who will tell me about the results?

Once your doctor is certain that you have asthma, you will talk about asthma and its treatment. Your job is to make sure you understand. Don't hesitate to ask the meaning of a word or to ask for more explanation. You might repeat what your doctor tells you to see if you've understood. Feel free to write down instructions and other information. You may not remember everything your doctor said during the visit. It's often helpful to read information when you get home. Be sure to ask for pamphlets, fact sheets, or names of current books that you can read and share with family members. Because you may think of more questions after you leave the office, ask your doctor for a good time to call. Some health care providers reserve a certain part of the day to return calls to their patients. Other offices have a nurse on staff who handles patients' calls.

Tailoring Your Treatment Plan

Together, you and health care provider will design a treatment plan that puts you on the road to good health. I like to keep treatment plans as simple as possible. The simpler the plan, the easier it is to follow. Because asthma varies from person to person, no one treatment plan works for everyone. You can expect to go through a trial-and-error process to figure out what works best for you. The goals of your treatment plan are to:

- prevent chronic and troublesome symptoms, such as coughing or breathlessness

- maintain normal or near-normal lung function
- maintain normal activity levels
- minimize—or better yet, prevent—repeated asthma
- attacks, emergency room visits, or hospitalizations avoid side effects from asthma medications

To meet these goals, your treatment plan will combine three features: (1) ways to find and avoid asthma triggers; (2) medications to control your asthma; and (3) a plan to monitor your asthma daily. This combined strategy can help you prevent asthma episodes—if you stick with it every day. Each feature is described separately in the next three chapters.

As time goes by, your treatment plan may need to change. If you find that you're uncomfortable with a part of your plan, talk to your doctor. Maybe you're worried about the safety of your medicine. Or perhaps you aren't sure how to use your peak-flow meter correctly. The sooner you discuss any concerns or questions with your health care provider, the better. It's easiest to control asthma symptoms when they first appear, or first appear to get worse. That's why it's essential that you and your doctor work closely. The last part of your treatment plan is to see your doctor regularly.

Follow-up Visits

Your asthma care continues after your diagnosis. Follow-up visits are an opportunity for you and your doctor to see how your treatment plan is working. In the beginning, you'll see your health care provider a lot—sometimes every few weeks. Be patient. It will take a while to fine-tune your medication and other parts of your treatment plan. Once your asthma is under control (and depending on your situation), you might have follow-up visits every 6 to 12 months to see if your treatment plan is still working.

During this early phase, continue to communicate with your doctor. Be honest about your progress: what works and what doesn't. Be clear so that your doctor has useful information to work with. If something has prevented you from getting treatment, say so. Are you satisfied with your treatment plan? During your follow-up visit, here are some questions your doctor may ask:

- How many days and/or nights in the past week have you had a cough, shortness of breath, wheezing, or a tight feeling in your chest?
- Do you perform peak-flow readings at home? (If yes, bring your peak-flow chart to your appointment.)
- How many days in the past week has asthma restricted your physical activity?
- Have you had any asthma attacks since your last visit?
- Have you had any unscheduled visits to a doctor—including the emergency room—since your last visit?
- How many puffs of your short-acting, inhaled beta$_2$ agonist (quick-relief medicine) do you use per day?
- How many short-acting, beta$_2$ agonist inhalers did you use over the past month?
- What questions or concerns would you like to discuss with your doctor?
- In your opinion, how well-controlled is your asthma (very well-controlled, somewhat controlled, not well-controlled)?
- How satisfied are you with your asthma care (very satisfied, somewhat satisfied, not satisfied)?

SUMMARY: WORKING WITH YOUR HEALTH CARE PROVIDER

- Your relationship with your health care provider is one of the most important aspects of managing your asthma. You should feel comfortable about raising any questions or concerns with your doctor.
- Whether you're seeing a new doctor or one you've seen before, prepare a list of questions and concerns before your appointment. Be ready to update your doctor.
- No single treatment plan works for everyone. Together, you and your doctor will fine-tune your treatment plan over time.
- Follow-up visits help you chart your progress with your treatment plan.

ACTION PLAN

Making the most of your partnership with your doctor will help you take charge of your asthma—and your overall health. This chapter has shown you how. You're now ready to take the next steps:

- If you haven't seen your doctor in more than a year, make an appointment.
- Start a list of questions and concerns for your next doctor's appointment.
- Ask yourself what else you can do to control your asthma.
- Review your treatment plan.

Chapter 3

Asthma-Proofing Your World

Like all people with asthma, your airways are especially sensitive to certain "triggers." Triggers are things in your environment that prompt the chain reaction leading to an asthma attack. In the presence of certain triggers where you live and work, airways swell, tighten up, and produce too much mucus. While it's not completely understood why the airways of people with asthma react this way, researchers have uncovered many of the culprits that set the airways off. Just as asthma symptoms differ from person to person, so do the triggers that bother each person.

Controlling your asthma, then, involves finding your personal asthma triggers. There are many common triggers. Sometimes, the suspected trigger reveals itself easily. Other times, you may have to do additional footwork to identify your triggers.

The goal of this chapter is to help you identify and avoid your personal triggers. I'll discuss some control measures that you can easily put into place at home and away from home. Be sure to enlist the help of your doctor in this endeavor. You and your doctor will figure out what actions you need to take first, discuss the results of your efforts, and see if other solutions might work better for you in your overall plan. Your asthma trigger control plan works together with your medicine plan, which is described in Chapter 4, "Asthma Medications."

If allergies trigger your asthma, you may be wondering about allergy testing and the value of allergy shots. These two topics are covered in this chapter, in the allergen section. Finally, you'll also find information about devices that affect the quality of indoor air and which ones are worth the investment.

You'll probably see a payoff from your quest quickly.

Your asthma symptoms may lessen, and you may see a drop-off in the number of asthma attacks. You may even be able to reduce the amount of medicine you need. You'll be surprised at how even small, easy changes can make a difference in the quality of your life.

Before we look at how to uncover asthma triggers, it's important to note that family members and coworkers can help you in your search. Because you live with your family and want their support, you might even ask one of them to go to the doctor's office with you. Your doctor can explain to them about your asthma triggers and the importance of avoiding them. Family members can then help you eliminate the triggers from your home. On the job, coworkers can also help you figure out what triggers your asthma symptoms and can help you asthma-proof your workplace.

LINING UP THE SUSPECTS

Fortunately, the triggers most likely to cause your airways to overreact have been implicated in many people with asthma. That means that you can start your search by considering these common triggers first. Chances are your personal triggers are the same.

Triggers fall into two categories: inhalant allergens (things that you breathe in that cause an allergic reaction) and irritants (things that increase airway inflammation and asthma symptoms without an allergic response). Irritants include cigarette smoke; infections; exercise; cold, dry weather; air pollution; strong odors or sprays; medications; and exposure to substances on the job. Allergen triggers include dust mites, cockroach droppings, pollen, and dander (I'll explain what dander is below).

Some of the allergens that trigger asthma are the same as those that trigger the sneezing, itchy or watery eyes, and runny or stuffy nose that we typically call "allergies." The medical term for these symtoms is allergic rhinitis (rhinitis literally means "inflammation of the nose"). You may have heard it referred to as "hay fever." Hay fever is a common term for allergic rhinitis caused by ragweed pollen. Allergic rhinitis may also be caused by pollen from various grasses and trees as well as other inhalant allergens.

If you have asthma that is triggered by allergens, your allergic reaction occurs mainly in your lungs. You get asthma symptoms instead of allergic rhinitis symptoms. Your airways may feel twitchy or ticklish, yet your nose, eyes, and throat are fine.

Allergies are the result of an inappropriate response by the body's immune system to an offending agent. However, it is only after the first exposure that your immune system "labels" something an offending agent or foreign invader. Allergic reactions happen only after a second or later contact with an allergen. Underlying an allergic response is a complex interaction of chemicals that are produced naturally by the body's immune system.

Basically, when you breathe in an allergen that you are sensitive to, your body responds to this invader by releasing chemicals called mediators. Histamine is one of these mediators. There are several steps in between, but let's keep things simple. The histamine makes the lining of the eyelids and eyes, sinuses, and nasal passages swell. If you have asthma, the response to the histamine occurs in your airways. Instead of sneezing, a runny nose, and itchy eyes, you may have an asthma attack. These allergic reactions are inherited. If someone in your family has allergies, the chance that you will too is increased.

Asking the Right Questions

The following questions will give you clues as to which triggers—both irritant and allergen—may be to blame:

- Is your asthma worse in certain months? If so, do your asthma symptoms appear at the same time as those of allergies? A yes answer means that you may be allergic to pollen or outdoor molds.
- Do your asthma symptoms appear when visiting a

house where there are indoor pets? If so, consider dander as the source. Dander is a substance found in some animal's hair, including those of cats and dogs—and even humans. Some people are highly allergic to dander.
- If you have pets in your home, do asthma symptoms, such as nasal, eye, and chest symptoms, lessen when you are away from home longer than a week? Do the symptoms worsen within the 24 hours after returning home? If so, consider dander as the source.
- Do your eyes itch and redden after handling your pet (or someone else's)? If yes, you may have an allergy to dander, which may trigger your asthma.
- Do asthma symptoms appear when carpets are vacuumed? If you answer yes, dander and house-dust mites may be the cause. Dust mites are extremely tiny "bugs" that thrive in house dust, particularly in humid climates. House dust comes from the breakdown of materials in the home, such as furniture, pillow stuffing, human skin flakes, carpeting, feathers and mold spores. Dust mites live where human dander collects, such as your mattress, bedding, furniture, and carpets. House-dust mites are so small that you can't see them.
- Does making a bed cause asthma symptoms? If yes, then you can point a finger at those house-dust mites.
- Do you have asthma symptoms around hay or in a barn or stable? Here, a yes answer means molds and mites are the triggers.
- Do your asthma symptoms appear when you go into a damp basement or a vacation cottage that has been closed up for long periods? If so, then molds may be your triggers.
- Do your asthma symptoms occur only when you perform certain job activities, either at work or after leaving work? If so, do your symptoms improve when away from work for a few days? If so, a trigger may exist in your workplace.
- Do your asthma symptoms appear when you are near any of the following: tobacco smoke; wood smoke; scented products, such as hair spray, cosmetics, and cleaning products; strong odors, such as that of fresh paint or cooking; or automobile fumes or other air

pollutants? Which ones? If any of these substances cause symptoms, they may be an asthma trigger.

Becoming Aware

What did you uncover by answering these questions? Did you see a connection between some of your asthma symptoms and certain triggers? You may find that you aren't aware of some of your triggers just yet. Fortunately, now that you know the patterns and suspects to look for, additional triggers will become apparent. The next step is to remove and avoid these triggers around the places you work and live as much as possible.

YOUR ASTHMA TRIGGER CONTROL PLAN

I've broken down the types of allergens and irritants into categories so that you can go directly to the ones that apply to you based on your responses to the above questions. Under each category, I've listed the actions you need to take to control your specific triggers. You can use these actions as a "To Do" list, checking off each step that you've completed.

Strategies for Allergens

Outdoor Pollens and Molds

Granted, you can't asthma-proof the great outdoors. However, you can limit your exposure to outdoor pollens and mold spores to reduce your asthma symptoms. If you have experienced asthma symptoms in early spring, tree pollens may be one of your asthma triggers; late spring, grasses; late summer to autumn, weeds; summer and fall, alternaria and cladosporium, both of which are molds.

- Stay inside in the middle of the day and afternoon, when the pollen and spore counts are highest.

- Exercise and do other outdoor activities just after sunrise, when pollen and spore counts are lowest.
- Use air conditioning, if possible.
- Close windows during seasons when pollen and mold are highest. Your health care provider can tell you when these seasons are in your area.
- Avoid wet leaves, yard debris, and other outdoor sources of mold.
- Avoid pillows, bedding, and furniture stuffed with kapok, a silky, fibrous material made from the seed pods of the silk-cotton tree. The fibers could contain pollen and spores.

House Dust Mite Control

House-dust mites depend on air moisture and human dander to survive. Mites occur in most areas of the United States. However, mites usually shun areas at high altitudes or dry areas, unless moisture is added to indoor air. In your home, your bed is the most important source of dust mites.

You may have seen products on the market designed to kill mites or make them less able to cause an allergic reaction. However, according to the guidelines issued in 1997 by the National Heart, Lung and Blood Institute, the effects are not dramatic or long-lasting. Routine use of these products is not recommended. Vacuuming does a good job at removing mite allergen from carpets but fails to remove live mites.

Here are some practical tips that have been shown to reduce the number of dust mites in your home:

- Encase your mattress and box spring in an airtight, allergen-impermeable cover. You can purchase these covers at department stores and other stores that sell bedding.
- Either encase your pillow in an airtight, allergen-impermeable cover or wash it once a week.
- Wash your bed covers, clothes, and stuffed toys once a week in hot water (130° Fahrenheit or higher, the temperature necessary for killing house-dust mites).

Finally, here are some things you can do that are worthwhile, but not essential, in controlling dust mites:

- Avoid sleeping or lying down on upholstered furniture.
- Remove carpets that are laid on concrete.
- Reduce indoor humidity to less than 50 percent. Use a dehumidifier if needed.
- Remove carpets from your bedroom.

Animal Allergens

There is no such thing as an allergen-free cat or dog. Nor does the type or length of a pet's hair matter. Since all warm-blooded pets, such as dogs, cats, birds, and rodents, produce dander, urine, feces, and saliva—all of which contain allergens—you are vulnerable if you are sensitive to animal allergens.

- Remove animal and products made of feathers (for example, down pillows) from your home.
- If you must have a pet, keep the pet out of your bedroom and keep the bedroom door closed at all times.
- Remove upholstered furniture and carpets from the home or keep the pet off them.
- Wash the pet weekly. Even cats can be trained to accept a bath. Ask your vet about the best way to bathe your cat.
- Avoid visits to friends or relatives with pets. If you must go, take asthma medications before visiting homes and other places where animals are present. Ask your doctor about which asthma medications you should take.
- Avoid products made with feathers, such as pillows and comforters.

Cockroach Allergen

Cockroaches have thrived through the ages and seem indifferent to even the cleanest of homes. The places most likely to have cockroaches are cities.

- Do not leave food out or garbage exposed.
- Use poison baits, boric acid, and roach traps. Chemical agents, such as roach sprays, can irritate asthma. If you do use chemical products to control roaches, have someone else spray while you are away. The home should be well-ventilated (keep windows open) and you should not return until a few hours after spraying.

Indoor Molds

Humidity and dampness provide a hospitable environment for mold to grow. Of course, if you live in a region of the country where it rains a lot or has humid summers, for example, you can't control the weather. But you can keep your house relatively mold-free. Kitchens, bathrooms, and basements are usually the moistest areas of your home so you should target your efforts there.

- Keep bathrooms, kitchens, and basements well ventilated.
- Clean bathrooms, kitchens, and basements regularly.
- Do not use humidifiers.
- Repair all leaks to prevent moisture build-up.
- Use a dehumidifier for damp basement areas. Set the humidity level for less than 50 percent but greater than 25 percent. Be sure to empty and clean the unit often. Check the manufacturer's instrctions for cleaning the unit.

Food Allergens

Most allergens that induce asthma symptoms are ones that you breathe in. Food is a less common cause. But if you experience asthma symptoms after eating processed potatoes, shrimp, or dried fruit or when drinking beer or wine, you may be sensitive to the sulfites present in these foods—although sulfite allergy is a rare asthma trigger. Sulfites are used to preserve foods and beverages. If your asthma seems to be triggered by sulfites, avoid food and beverage products that contain these preservatives, and read ingredient labels before eating processed foods.

What about Allergy Testing and Shots?

Your health care provider may recommend allergy skin tests for you, especially if you have found it difficult to pinpoint the allergens to which you are sensitive. An allergist, a physician who specializes in treating allergies, can perform these relatively simple tests.

There are two ways to perform these tests. In one method, the allergist makes a small scratch on your skin, either on your arm or back. On this scratch, he or she will then put a drop of liquid containing an allergen. Often, you are tested with several common allergens that you are likely to be exposed to in the home or in your region of the country. Each allergen comes in its own liquid and requires a separate scratch. After a few minutes, you may notice a red, itchy bump (hive) at the scratch site on which the allergen was placed. This reaction suggests that you are allergic to that particular allergen. In the second method, the allergist may simply give you an injection of the allergen and watch for a reaction at the injection site. Each allergen, again, requires a separate injection.

With the results of these skin tests, you can asthma-proof your home and take steps to avoid these allergens. Combined with your medication and the rest of your asthma management plan, you'll find that you can decrease the number of asthma attacks. In some instances, your doctor may recommend immunotherapy. You may know immunotherapy by its more common name, allergy shots. In the guidelines issued by the National Heart, Lung and Blood Institute in 1997, the expert panel recommended that physicians should consider immunotherapy for people whose asthma symptoms are poorly controlled by medications and are caused by allergens that are impossible to avoid or that occur for a major portion of the year or all year.

Immunotherapy decreases your response to the particular allergens that were identified by your allergy skin tests. You receive injections containing tiny amounts of the allergens, typically a few times a month for a three- to five-year period. With each injection, the percentage of the allergen is increased. Over time, the body's reaction to that allergen lessens.

Immunotherapy is not as widely used as it once was. In many studies, immunotherapy has proven to have little or no effect on alleric asthma. Furthermore, immunotherapy may cause a serious reaction, especially bronchoconstriction, more frequently among people with asthma (from 5 to 35 percent) compared with people who have allergic rhinitis. However, these reactions are rare. Allergy shots may also cause a severe, life-threatening allergic response called anaphylactic shock. Although anaphylactic shock is also rare, you should get your allergy shots in the doctor's office where the staff is prepared to deal with anaphylactic shock. For all of these reasons, be sure to discuss its risks and benefits with your doctor if you are considering immunotherapy.

Dealing with Irritants

Tobacco Smoke

Tobacco smoke is a major trigger of asthma symptoms. But your asthma is not the only reason to avoid tobacco smoke. Tobacco smoke and secondhand tobacco smoke are harmful to your health. Heart disease, cancer, and emphysema have all been linked to tobacco use.

- Do not smoke. If you do smoke, quit. Your doctor can help you quit or recommend programs. Local chapters of the American Heart Association and the American Lung Association can direct you to smoking cessation classes in your area or provide you with reading materials that can guide you on kicking the habit on your own. You might also check local hospitals for classes.
- Ask household members and visitors to smoke outside.
- Encourage household members to quit smoking.

Wood Smoke

Burning logs in the fireplace can mean trouble for a person with asthma whose airways are sensitive to wood smoke. To warm your house, you'll have to turn to gas, oil, or electric heat.

- Avoid using a wood-burning stove to heat your home.
- Do not use kerosene heaters.
- Avoid exposure to fumes from unvented gas, oil, or kerosene stoves and wood-burning appliances or fireplaces.

Strong Odors and Sprays

While some odors may smell pleasant, you may find that strong odors and sprays—even ones that smell nice—are the cause of your asthma symptoms. These days, you can find more and more products that are available in fragrance-free versions.

- Leave your home while it is being painted. Return to your house once the paint has dried.
- Avoid perfume and perfumed products, including talcum powder and hairspray. Opt for fragrance-free products.
- Do not use room deodorizers.
- Use fragrance-free household cleaning products.
- Use a fan or open windows in the kitchen to reduce cooking odors.
- Avoid exposure to air pollution by remaining inside on days when pollution is high.

Other Triggers

Weather. Temperature changes, humidity, wind, and barometric pressure have also been implicated in triggering asthma. If you notice that these weather conditions cause you to have asthma symptoms, some strategies can help. For example, cover your mouth and nose with a scarf or turtleneck on cold or windy days. On humid days, head indoors and use a dehumidifier.

Exercise. About 85 percent of people with allergic asthma wheeze after exercise. Breathing in cool, dry air may be the trigger. You may find that some forms of exercise, such as swimming, do not cause asthma symptoms. It is possible to stay active—and even be an Olympic athlete—even if you have asthma. You can read more about exercise-induced asthma in Chapter 6, "Living with Asthma: Special Types of Asthma."

Occupational Irritants. Workplace exposure to fumes, vapors, chemicals, and dusts can bring on asthma symptoms, usually several hours after you have been on the job. Occupational asthma is sometimes hard to pinpoint. It may take awhile for you to see a connection between your asthma attacks and the workplace. I discuss occupational asthma and how to deal with it in greater detail in Chapter 6.

Medications. Aspirin and other nonsteroidal anti-inflammatory drugs (NSAIDS) and certain beta blockers (so-called nonselective types) may trigger an asthma attack. NSAIDS include ibuprofen (known by the trade names Advil and Motrin), indomethacin (Indocin), and naproxen sodium (Aleve, Anaprox). Nonselective beta blockers, such as those found in eye drops for treatment of glaucoma, have been shown to cause asthma symptoms and should also be avoided. When taking any prescription or nonprescription medication, be sure to ask your health care provider or pharmacist whether it contains aspirin or other NSAIDS or beta blockers. If you have experienced a reaction to NSAIDS, do not take them. Use acetaminophen instead.

DEVICES THAT AFFECT INDOOR AIR

Numerous devices are available that may or may not improve the quality of indoor air. Some of them are expensive yet don't live up to the manufacturer's promise. New products come out every year that claim to reduce or eliminate airborne allergens and irritants. My advice to you? *Caveat emptor.* It's a Latin saying meaning, "Let the buyer beware." If a device sounds too good to be true, then it probably is. Only a few devices have been proven effective for modifying indoor air.

Here is some information about the various devices on the market that you may be tempted to buy to help reduce your asthma symptoms. As you'll see, not all devices are effective in controlling asthma, although some are.

Vacuum cleaners

Use a vacuum cleaner fitted with a HEPA (high-efficiency particulate air) filter or with a double bag. HEPA filters are expensive but do the job well. Do not fall for advertising claims for other types of filters. Conventional vacuum cleaners aren't helpful. You might also buy a central vacuum cleaner that has the collecting bag outside of your home. You should stay out of rooms where a vacuum cleaner is being used or has just been used. Vacuuming stirs up the particles that make up house dust. If you must vacuum, wear a dust mask.

Humidifiers and evaporative (swamp) coolers

These devices are not recommended for use in the homes of people who are sensitive to house-dust mites. They both increase humidity, which may encourage the growth of dust mites and mold. Additionally, humidifiers that are not properly cleaned can house and spread mold spores.

Air conditioning

Air conditioning allows you to keep windows and doors closed during warm weather—critical if you are allergic to outdoor pollens and molds. Regular use of central air conditioning will help keep humidity in check, which may also decrease house dust mite population and growth of mold.

Dehumidifiers

If you live in areas of the country where the humidity is high for most of the year, consider investing in a dehumidifier. By keeping household humidity levels low, a dehumidifier will also help reduce house-dust mite and mold growth.

Indoor air-cleaning devices

These devices are not a substitute for asthma trigger control strategies listed earlier. In fact, those strategies are more effective at curbing asthma triggers. HEPA and electrostatic precipitating filters may reduce airborne cat dander, mold spores, and tobacco smoke. However, these filters cannot reduce your exposure to heavy particles, such as house dust mite and cockroach allergens, because they do not remain in the air.

Air duct cleaning of heating, ventilation, air conditioning systems

Cleaning of household air ducts may decrease airborne mold in your home. However, no studies have been done to examine the effect on levels of house dust mite or dander.

IF YOU NEED A PLAN B

Problems with avoiding triggers? Take advantage of the partnership you've successfully built with your doctor. (For a quick review, look over Chapter 2, "Working With Your Health Care Provider.") Talk to your doctor and explain what and why you are having a problem in avoiding or eliminating exposures to the triggers you've identified. Let him or her know what solutions you have tried, what worked, and what didn't. With your input, your health care provider can work with you and your family in finding practical solutions and compromises that will help you eliminate triggers.

Asthma-proofing your world is one way that you can

control your asthma. Time and time again, I have seen how effective these steps are. My own daughter needed convincing that dust mites in bedding might be a problem. When she saw that coughing at night went away after she followed the steps outlined in this chapter, she was a believer. Your trigger control plan works hand-in-hand with your medication plan, which is the topic of the next chapter.

SUMMARY

- Asthma triggers cause your airways to swell, tighten up, and produce too much mucus. Identifying your own triggers that cause asthma attacks can help you control your asthma. Your doctor can help you figure out what your triggers are and how to asthma-proof your world.
- Asthma triggers fall into two categories: irritants and inhalant allergens. Weather, exercise, and some medications can also cause asthma symptoms.
- Allergy skin tests can help you pinpoint inhalant allergens that trigger your asthma. In certain instances, your physician may recommend immunotherapy, or allergy shots.
- Only a few indoor-air cleaning devices have been proven effective for modifying indoor air. If a manufacturer's claims sound too good to be true, then they probably are. Use a vacuum cleaner with a HEPA filter. Avoid using humidifiers, but air conditioners and dehumidifiers are helpful. Talk to your doctor before buying any devices.

ACTION PLAN

With all of the information you have learned in this chapter, you are ready to:

- Review your asthma trigger control plan. What do I need to do now? Is there anything more I can do?
- Monitor your asthma, as described in Chapter 5, be-

fore and after you put your asthma trigger control plan into place. Is it working?
- Make a list of questions and concerns about your asthma trigger control plan before your next doctor's appointment. Discuss your asthma trigger control plan with your doctor. Ask him or her for help when you are having trouble identifying or avoiding triggers.
- Enlist household members and coworkers to help you uncover triggers and asthma-proof your environment.
- Read Chapter 4, "Asthma Medications," and Chapter 5, "Managing Your Asthma Day to Day." These chapters have information that will work hand-in-hand with your asthma trigger control plan.

Chapter 4

Asthma Medications

No matter what triggers your asthma, medicine can help you control it. This chapter will explain these medications. As you read, you'll learn what to expect from your medication, the major types of asthma medicine, how you and your doctor decide on a medicine plan, techniques for inhaling medication, and how to make the most of your medicine as time goes by. At the end of the chapter, I also include a few important points to discuss with your doctor.

WHAT TO EXPECT FROM ASTHMA MEDICATION

You might be wondering why you need asthma medication in the first place. Maybe you're bothered by a wheezy cough, but you buy over-the-counter medicine to treat it. Or perhaps you've read about people with asthma who found relief in a new diet, relaxation therapy, or even acupuncture. Some of these approaches might work some of the time. But the truth is that none of them come close to the power of prescription medication. Asthma is a unique condition, and researchers have developed a range of drugs designed specifically to treat it.

In the first few chapters of this book, you learned that your asthma—from symptoms to triggers—is different from anyone else's. So is the medication that can help. When you first learn about the many kinds of prescription asthma medicine, you may feel a little overwhelmed. That's normal. There are a lot of choices. But don't panic. Working together, you and your doctor can create a "medicine plan" that helps you breathe easier every day. You'll begin by trying one or several medications. Depending on how your asthma responds, your medicine plan may change. By carefully monitoring your medication and your symptoms, you'll find the right combination of drugs to treat your asthma. When your medicine plan is working, you can expect:

- Fewer asthma attacks
- Little chronic coughing or breathing problems, even at night
- Fewer emergency trips to the doctor or hospital
- Freedom to be active, including exercise

A NOTE ABOUT OVER-THE-COUNTER ASTHMA MEDICINE

Most asthma medications are only available with your doctor's prescription. A few inhaled quick-reliever medications, however, are sold over-the-counter at drugstores. These general medications are advertised to treat asthma, chronic bronchitis, emphysema, and other lung disease. Don't use them. As you've learned, everyone's asthma is different. Together, you and your doctor can decide which—and how much—medication is right for you. Simply puffing on an over-the-counter inhaler whenever you feel short of breath will not improve your asthma. And it may even make your symptoms worse.

MAJOR TYPES OF ASTHMA MEDICATION

When you think of asthma, you probably think of asthma attacks, which are short bouts of wheezing and breathing problems. But asthma is more than just the occasional attack. It's a chronic (lasting) disease that causes your lungs to remain swollen, or inflamed, all the time. To fight both asthma attacks and the chronic inflammation of asthma, doctors use two types of medicine, quick relievers and long-term controllers. In the following section, I present a brief review of the major drugs currently being used to treat asthma.

Quick Relievers

Quick-relief medications help stop an asthma attack after it has begun. These drugs work by relaxing the muscles that tighten in and around your bronchial tubes, or airways, during an attack. For this reason, they're called bronchodilators. If you have mild asthma (brief asthma attacks only once or twice a week), a quick reliever may be the only medication you need.

Quick relievers include:

- Short-acting beta$_2$ agonists
- Theophylline

Short-acting Beta$_2$ Agonists

Short-acting beta$_2$ agonists are the most common quick relievers. They work by stimulating the nerves that relax the muscles around the airways. When you're having an asthma attack, you can take a beta$_2$ agonist to help stop the attack. These drugs include albuterol (brand names: Proventil, Ventolin), pirbuterol acetate (Maxair), terbutaline sulfate (Brethaire), bitolterol mesylate (Tornalate), and metaproterenol sulfate (Alupent, Metrapel).

How do you take a beta$_2$ agonist? During an asthma attack, you breathe in a beta$_2$ agonist using an inhaler. The medication travels to your lungs and begins working to relax your airways within minutes. Short-acting beta$_2$ agonists can help keep your asthma symptoms at bay for about 4 hours.

When do you take a beta$_2$ agonist? Your doctor will tell you to use a short-acting beta$_2$ agonist on an "as-needed" basis, or whenever you're having a hard time breathing. Keep in mind that you should only use a beta$_2$ agonist 2 or 3 times a week. If you find yourself needing your inhaler more often than this, call your doctor. Your medication isn't controlling your asthma, and you may need to try another kind of drug.

What are the side effects? In general, short-acting beta$_2$

agonists cause few side effects. These effects may include a faster heart beat, tremors, an anxious feeling, and a sick stomach or nausea. Rarely, more serious side effects occur, including chest pain, a dizzy feeling, vomiting, bad headaches, or a very fast heart beat. If you have any of these symptoms, call your doctor immediately. Finally, you must be aware that the overuse of short-acting beta$_2$ agonists may cause a "rebound" effect, which can make asthma worse.

Theophylline

Theophyllie is another type of quick reliever. Theophylline (brand names: Theo-Dur, Respbid, Slo-Bid, Theo-24, Theolair, Uniphyl, Slo-Phyllin) is not used as commonly as the beta$_2$ agonists. It takes longer to work, so it does not help as quickly during an acute asthma attack. Some people find taking theophylline at bedtime helps them breathe better throughout the night, when asthma symptoms often get worse. Like all quick relievers, theophylline relaxes the muscles around the airways. However, researchers still aren't sure how theophylline accompishes this effect.

How do you take theophylline? This medication comes in liquid, tablet, or capsule form.

When do you take theophylline? Your doctor may tell you to take theophylline every 8 or 12 hours. It's best to take this medication with food. Because theophylline's effect gradually builds in your body, it's important to take your medicine on time. If you miss a dose, however, do not take twice as much the next time. This medication is too strong. Instead, take the normal amount and check with your doctor about any missed medicine.

What are the side effects? If you take low doses of theophylline, your side effects should be minimal. You might feel like you do after drinking coffee. Like caffeine, theophylline can make you feel nervous, unable to sleep, or sick to your stomach. The higher the dose of the drug, the worse these symptoms may be. In some rare cases, the drug can cause seizures. Talk to your doctor before taking theophylline if you have high blood pressure, peptic ulcer disease, or any heart condition.

What To Remember About Quick Relievers

Don't Overuse Them. If you need to use a quick-reliever medicine often, it may be a sign that the swelling in your airways is getting worse. It also may mean your medication isn't working properly. If you need a short-acting beta$_2$ agonist at least 3 times a week, see your doctor. You may need to take a controller medication every day, while using a quick reliever just during asthma attacks. (One exception to the no-more-than-3-times-a-week rule is exercise-induced asthma. If you are an athlete with asthma, ask your doctor how often to take asthma medication.)

Technique Matters. No matter what your asthma symptoms, your doctor probably will suggest that you keep an inhaler nearby in case you need a quick reliever medication during an asthma attack. To get the full benefit of these drugs, you must use the right inhaler technique. I'll discuss how to use inhalers later in this chapter.

Long-Term Controllers

Long-term-controller medications help keep your asthma in check every day. These drugs work by reducing the chronic swelling, or inflammation, in your lungs. For this reason, they're called anti-inflammatory medications. Long-term controllers basically calm your airways, leaving your lungs less prone to asthma attacks. In recent years, doctors have discovered just how important controller medications are. If you have moderate-to-severe asthma (attacks twice or more a week), your health care provider will prescribe a controller.

Long-term controllers include:

- Corticosteroids
- Cromolyn sodium and nedocromil sodium
- Long-acting beta$_2$ agonists
- Leukotriene antagonists

Corticosteroids

Corticosteroids are the most common type of long-term controllers. These drugs act to decrease the acticity of a variety of cells that lead to inflammation in your lungs. Today's inhaled corticosteroids include beclomethasone dipropionate (brand names: Beclovent, Vanceril), dexamethasone sodium phosphate (Decadron Phosphate Respihaler), triamcinolone acetonide (Azmacort), and flunisolide (AeroBid, AeroBid-M). Oral (pill, tablet, or liquid) corticosteroids include prednisone (brand names: Deltasone, Liquid Pred, Metocorten, Orasone, Panasol, Prednicen-M, Sterapred) and prednisolone (Pediapred, Medrol).

How do you take a corticosteroid? If your doctor thinks you need a corticosteroid, he or she will suggest that you try an inhaled corticosteroid. Like any inhaled asthma medication, it goes directly to your lungs, working just where it's needed. Sometimes, however, you might benefit from an oral corticosteroid. Oral corticosteroids are "systemic" drugs: they travel throughout your body. Because systemic corticosteroids are so potent, they quickly reduce your lung inflammation. Once your asthma symptoms are under control, you will likely switch to the inhaled variety.

When do you take a corticosteroid? Because an inhaled corticosteroid constantly works to reduce lung swelling, it's very important that you take this drug every day, even when you feel fine. If you have moderate asthma, your doctor will probably suggest you start by inhaling 2 to 4 puffs once a day. This dosage can vary, however, and it may change depending on how your asthma responds. For oral corticosteroids, your doctor will determine the dosage that's right for you.

What are the side effects? When used at the recommended dosage, inhaled corticosteroids have few side effects in adults. Potential side effects include yeast infections in the mouth, loss of voice or hoarseness, and coughing. You usually can avoid these problems by learning the right inhaler technique.

High doses of inhaled corticosteroids may, in some people, increase the risk of osteoporosis (weakening of the bones) and ulcers and may cause easy bruising or skin conditions. If your child has asthma, talk to your doctor about the right dosage of inhaled corticosteroids. Some studies suggest these drugs can, over a long period, lead to a slightly delayed growth in children. However, asthma appears to do this as well. Your doctor can explain the risks and benefits of asthma medication.

Oral corticosteroids cause more side effects than the inhaled variety. That's why these drugs are typically used for only a short time, usually 3 to 10 days. During short-term use, systemic corticosteroids may temporarily cause weight gain, increased appetite, mood alteration, high blood pressure, or peptic ulcers. Taken over a long period of time, these systemic drugs may sometimes lead to delayed growth in children, diabetes, cataracts, muscle weakness, skin problems, and other conditions. Many of these complications, however, can be avoided by certain medication schedules—for example, taking the drugs every other day, rather than every day. Talk to your health care provider about how to avoid side effects when taking oral corticosteroids.

Cromolyn Sodium and Nedocromil Sodium

These anti-inflammatory drugs are sometimes used instead of, or in addition to, corticosteroids to treat mild, persistent asthma (at least one attack every week, with occasional coughing, wheezing, or other symptoms). Cromolyn is sold as Intal; nedocromil as Tilade. Both drugs may help prevent asthma attacks caused by allergies, exercise, or cold air. If you know you'll soon be near a substance—dander, for example—that triggers your asthma, you might take one of these drugs ahead of time. You might also take one before exercising, if you tend to feel wheezy afterward.

How do you take cromolyn or nedocromil? Both these drugs are inhaled.

When do you take these drugs? That depends on your asthma. Your doctor may suggest taking 1 or 2 puffs of cromolyn or nedocromil a day, or before you go near certain asthma triggers.

What are the side effects? These drugs have very few side effects. Because of its safety, cromolyn is often prescribed for children. In 1997, nedocromil also was approved for use by children 6 years of age and older. Either drug may be added to a medicine plan rather than simply increasing the dosage of corticosteroids. A small number of people report getting a bad taste in their mouth from nedocromil.

Long-Acting Beta$_2$ Agonists

Like short-acting beta$_2$ agonists (see "Quick Relievers," above), these drugs help relax your airways. But they act over a longer period of time. The drugs can be convenient because a little bit goes a long way. If you're using an inhaled corticosteroid but still have some asthma symptoms, a long-acting beta$_2$ agonist may help you become symptom-free. These drugs, which are relatively new, include salmeterol, sold under the brand name Serevent.

How do you take a long-acting beta$_2$ agonist? Salmeterol is inhaled.

When do you take these drugs? Because these drugs keep your airways relaxed for around 12 hours, they're often used at bedtime. If you normally wake up wheezing during the night, you might try a long-acting beta$_2$ agonist before you go to sleep. You also might take these drugs a half-hour before exercising, if you normally have an asthma attack afterward. Use these drugs no more than twice a day (about 4 puffs on an inhaler per day). Also, note that long-acting beta$_2$ agonists cannot help you during an acute asthma attack. Do not take them. Instead, use a short-acting quick reliever.

What are the side effects? Taken once or twice a day, long-acting beta$_2$ agonists appear to cause few side effects. Shakiness, higher blood pressure, headaches, or a faster heart beat are possible. Over time, some people who use salmeterol every day may find the drug stops working as well. Because long-acting beta$_2$ agonists are relatively new, researchers still are studying their long-term effects.

Tips For Taking Long-Acting Beta$_2$ Agonists: These drugs do *not* replace your other controller medications. Even when you feel fine, do not stop taking your daily medicine. And never take a long-acting beta$_2$ agonist during an asthma attack. It will not stop your attack. Reach for a short-acting quick reliever instead.

Leukotriene Antagonists

First available in 1996, these controller medications work by blocking leukotrienes, a class of mediators in the body that contribute to lung inflammation in people with asthma. Because these drugs are so new, we are still learning their role in asthma management. Leukotriene antagonists appear to help adults with mild to moderate asthma. If you are taking a low-dose inhaled corticosteroid but still have some asthma symptoms, your health care provider may suggest adding a leukotriene modifier. This combination may keep you from needing a quick reliever (see above) medication several times a week. A handful of leukotriene antagonists are in development. The first to reach market were zafirlukast (brand name: Accolate) and zileuton (Zyflo).

How do you take a leukotriene antagonist? Zafirlukast and zileuton both come as tablets.

When do you take a leukotriene antagonist? Like most controllers, you take a leukotriene modifier every day. How often you take it each day depends on the drug. Zileuton, for example, is taken 4 times a day; Zafirlukast, just twice a day.

What are the side effects? Depending on the exact drug, leukotriene antagonists have different side effects. Most of these effects are mild. Zileuton may cause an upset stomach. In some people, the drug may affect liver function. Zafirlukast may sometimes cause headaches, nausea, or certain infections. Talk to your doctor about ways to limit these side effects.

What To Remember About Long-Term Controllers

Take Them Every Day. It's very important that you take these drugs every day—even if you feel fine. If you don't take your controller medicine, the muscles in your airways may begin to swell without you knowing it. That leaves you vulnerable to more—and more severe—asthma attacks. It's easy to forget to take daily medication. But it's worth it to remember. In one study, patients who used their controller medications every day soon stopped needing to take quick-reliever drugs all the time. Their lung function improved. They also visited the doctor less.

They Take Time To Work. Unlike with quick-reliever medications, your asthma symptoms will not immediately respond to a long-term controller. These drugs begin to work gradually in your body. When you begin taking a daily inhaled corticosteroid, for example, several days may pass before you notice that you're breathing more easily. So even if you don't feel better yet, it's important to keep taking your medication as prescribed. If you think your medicine isn't working, talk to your doctor. Over time, you will learn how to increase or decrease the dosage of some medications.

What To Remember About All Asthma Medications

Asthma Medicine Is Safe. Any type of medication can cause some side effects. But remember that asthma medicine, taken at the recommended doses and times, is safe for most people. Your doctor can explain the risks and benefits of your medicine. Ask about side effects, about using other medications at the same time, and about your current and past health conditions. It's important that you feel comfortable with your medicine plan.

Tell Your Doctor About Other Drugs and Health Conditions. A few types of medication can react with asthma drugs. If you are being treated for high blood pressure, heart problems, or migraine headaches, your medication might make your asthma worse. These conditions are sometimes treated with drugs called beta-blockers, which may interfere with asthma medication. The same is true for aspirin. If you are taking any medication at all, tell your doctor before you begin your asthma medicine plan. Also, if you have any existing health conditions—if you are pregnant, for example—let your health care provider know.

Different Medications Work For Different People. The asthma medications that work so well for your best friend may not work for you. You may need to try several types (and amounts) of medicine before you find the right combination. If you have moderate or severe asthma, your doctor will recommend both long-term controller and quick-reliever drugs. Also, keep in mind that different medications may be appropriate for young adults, elderly adults, and children. In Chapter 9, I'll address asthma in the young and old.

New Drugs Are On The Horizon. Asthma drugs will continue to improve. Drug companies are constantly developing new medications that work better, last longer, and cause fewer side effects than existing drugs. Phosphodiesterase inhibitors (PDE4 inhibitors), for example, like theopylline but without the side effects. These drugs act to stop natural chemicals in the body that lead to lung inflammation. PDE4 inhibitors should be available in coming years. Always ask your doctor about the latest medications available.

YOUR MEDICINE PLAN: GETTING STARTED

With all these choices, how do you get started on a medicine plan? Your first step is diagnosis. Asthma is not the same for everyone. Some people have short asthma attacks once a week. Others have bouts of wheezing several times a day. The medication that's best for you largely depends on how frequent and severe your asthma symptoms are. In general, there are three basic levels of asthma: mild, moderate, and severe.

If you have *mild asthma*, you get brief attacks just once or twice a week. Your asthma symptoms may be intermittent (bothering you just occasionally) or *persistent*, affecting you even between attacks. Your breathing, as measured by a peak-flow meter, is about 80 percent as effective as it should be. (Peak-flow meters are discussed in Chapter 5, "Managing Your Asthma Day to Day"). Your breathing ability is about the same during day and night. If you this description fits you, your health care provider will probably suggest you inhale a short-acting beta$_2$ agonist during your asthma attacks. This quick-reliever medication should help you breathe easier in a matter of minutes. You may also need to keep track of your daily breathing patterns by using a peak flow-meter at home.

If you have *moderate asthma*, you often get asthma attacks more than twice a week. Your attacks may involve more serious coughing, wheezing, and breathing problems. Your breathing ability, as measured by peak flow rate, is 60–80 percent of what's normal. You have a harder time breathing at night. If this description fits you, your health care provider may recommend taking an inhaled corticosteroid (a long-term controller) every day and a short-acting beta$_2$ agonist (a quick reliever) during asthma attacks. You'll need to use a peak-flow meter at home to learn how much your breathing improves with this medication.

If you have *severe asthma,* you have an asthma attack almost every day. You also may have a chronic cough. You wake up at night because you can't breathe well. Your breathing ability, as measured by a peak-flow meter, may be about half of what it should be. If this description fits you, your doctor may suggest using a higher dosage of an inhaled corticosteroid (a long-term controller) every day and a short-acting beta$_2$ agonist (a quick reliever) during asthma attacks. Again, you'll want to use a peak-flow meter at home to track your breathing ability.

Keep in mind that the above descriptions are general. Remember, each person's asthma is different. You and your doctor will look at your individuals symptoms and decide which category you fall into.

Step-Down or Step-Up Approach?

All doctors share one basic goal for asthma management: to help you gain control of your asthma using as little medication as possible. This goal makes good health sense. While asthma medicines are safe, any drug can sometimes cause side effects. So we always want to use only the medications that are absolutely needed.

In keeping with this goal, many doctors are changing the way they treat asthma. We have learned that it's important to hit asthma hard at first and then gradually decrease medication to the lowest amount possible. This so-called "step-down" approach to therapy works to quickly get asthma symptoms under control. In 1997, the National Heart, Lung, and Blood Institute (NHLBI), a government agency that funds and conducts medical research, issued comprehensive guidelines to help doctors better diagnose and treat asthma. NHLBI encouraged doctors to try step-down care.

How does step-down care work? Using the classifications mentioned above, your health care provider first decides whether you have mild, moderate, or severe asthma. (Even within these grades, remember, asthma symptoms can vary.) Then, you will begin a course of medication to treat asthma that's one step "worse" than yours. For example, you may take an oral, or systemic, corticosteroid for a short time. This drug can quickly decrease the inflammation in your lungs. Once your lungs have improved, you would "step down" to less medication, such as a low-dose daily inhaled corticosteroid. This controller medication, then, would maintain your lungs' healthier state.

Some doctors still prefer the traditional "step-up" approach to asthma medication. In this approach, you begin your medicine plan using the least amount of medication possible. If your symptoms do not improve, your health care provider may suggest taking more or different kinds of medication.

No matter how you start your medicine plan starts, these first steps are critical. Now is the time for you to take control of your asthma. As you begin a medicine plan, you'll have regular follow-up visits with your doctor. Together, you will see how your asthma responds to medication. Is it improving? You may need less medicine. Is your breathing getting worse? Maybe you need a different medication. It's important for you to work closely with your health care provider. Partnership is the key to understanding your asthma and maintaining your health, today and for the years to come.

5 Tips To A Good Medicine Plan

As you begin your medicine plan, some tips may help.

Ask questions. Asthma medicine is complicated, and it's easy to get lost in the details. Can't remember the difference between a bronchodilator and an anti-inflammatory? Ask your doctor. Are you worried your medicine isn't safe or working right? Again, just ask. What about cost? Will your health insurance cover this medicine? Ask. Your doctor has most of the answers.

Write it down. Your health care provider may have worksheets that help you keep track of your medication. If not, ask for help in writing out your medicine plan. For each medication you take, ask your doctor these questions (and write down the answers):

- What's the name of this medication?
- What does it do? Is it a quick reliever or a long-term controller?
- When do I take it?
- How much do I take?
- Are there special instructions for taking this medicine?
- What if I miss a dose?
- Can I take other medications at the same time?
- Are there side effects I should expect or report?
- When do I (or can I) stop taking this medicine?

Simplify. When you're first starting a medicine plan, ask your health care provider to help you keep it simple. It can be confusing to take pills in the morning, inhale medicine in the afternoon, and take different pills at night. Whenever possible, create an easy medication schedule.

Try. The only person who can take your medication, learn inhaler technique, and measure your daily breathing patterns is you. Ask family members and friends for their encouragement. When you take your medication, avoid asthma triggers, and monitor your health, you'll breathe and feel better.

Stay flexible. Asthma changes from day to day, and your medical needs change with it. Over time, you may need to switch medications or change your dosage. The key to these transitions is being flexible. Stay on top of your asthma. If you seem to be improving—or getting worse—give your doctor a call.

HOW TO INHALE MEDICATION

Most of the time, the best way to take asthma medication is to inhale it. Inhaled medication goes right to your lungs and begins working quickly. As a result, it's usually faster and safer than oral (liquid or pill) medicine. When you inhale a beta$_2$ agonist during an asthma attack, for example, you should begin breathing better within about 10 minutes.

By comparison, a pill or liquid medication can take 1 to 3 hours to begin working. Because inhaled medicine acts only on your lungs, it also causes fewer side effects than oral drugs, which travel in your bloodstream all over your body. Both types of asthma medicine—quick relievers and long-term controllers—usually can be inhaled.

Most people with asthma use a metered dose inhaler (MDI) to inhale medication. An MDI is a small canister of medicine, much like a small spray can, that fits into a holder with a mouthpiece. When you push on the inhaler, it delivers a certain (metered) dose of medicine as a light spray or mist. Adults and children ages 5 and older can use MDIs. As an alternative, you might use a dry powder inhaler (DPI) or a nebulizer. Each of these devices is discussed below.

Learning to use an inhaler is one of the most important things you can do to control your asthma. When you inhale medication correctly, you get the full amount of that medication and send it directly to the lungs, where it does the most good. But when you use an inhaler improperly—breathing in too fast, for example—only some of the medicine reaches your lungs. If you are inhaling a long-term controller medication, your asthma will not improve (and it could get worse). If you are inhaling a quick reliever, your lungs may still get plenty of medication, but so could your mouth, the back of your throat, and the air around you. It's a lot more effective to send the medication just where it needs to go.

According to the American Lung Association, more than half of people who use inhalers do so incorrectly. It's easy to see why. Learning inhaler technique takes time, patience, and practice. If you follow a few simple steps, however, you can do it. As in all your asthma treatment, you have a helpful partner: your doctor. When you first get your inhaler, your doctor (or a nurse) will show you how it works. While in your doctor's office, practice using the inhaler. Also, ask for written instructions that you can review at home. It's easy to forget just when to inhale or how long to hold your breathe, even if you did it perfectly in the doctor's office. Written reminders can help. (Many organizations listed in Chapter 11, "For More Information," also offer inhaler tips.) Then, each time you visit your doctor for a check-up, bring your inhaler and practice with it again. Together, you can be sure you're doing everything right. You'll feel more confident and you'll control your asthma better, too.

Using a Metered Dose Inhaler (MDI)

Each time you use an inhaler, follow these steps (see Figure A):

1. Take off the cap and hold the inhaler upright.
2. Shake the inhaler.
3. Tilt your head back slightly and breathe out slowly.
4. Hold the inhaler about 2 inches in front of your mouth. Don't place the inhaler in your mouth.
5. At the same time, press down the inhaler and begin to breathe in slowly.
6. Continue to breathe in slowly for up to 5 seconds. It's important to inhale slowly and evenly, not sharply.
7. Hold your breath for 10 seconds. This lets the medicine travel deep into your lungs.
8. Repeat with another puff, if prescribed. If you wait

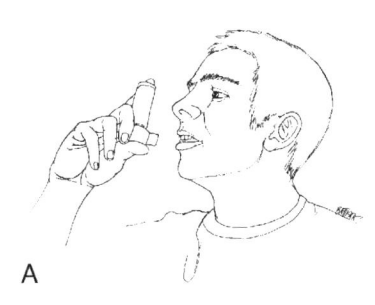

A

a minute or two between puffs, the medication may do a better job of reaching your lungs.

9. If you are inhaling two medications at once, it's best to inhale a quick reliever first, followed by a long-term controller.

Figure B shows an alternative way to inhale medication. Try the above way first. If you have trouble, try the way shown in Figure B.

Common Inhaler Mistakes

The above steps sound easy to do. But if you've tried it, you know that using an inhaler takes practice. People often make several mistakes. The major one is failing to breathe in and press down the inhaler at exactly the same time. Another problem is inhaling too fast. You also might forget to hold your breath long enough (up to 10 seconds) after inhaling the medicine. These mistakes can cause excess medicine to end up on your tongue, in the back of your throat, or just out in the air. You may cough, get a bad taste in your mouth, or, with corticosteroids, run an increased risk of developing oral infections.

Spacers

One solution to these problems is to use a spacer. A spacer is a holding device, shaped a bit like a big straw, that fits between the inhaler and your mouth. Spacers make inhaling asthma medicine easier. You close your lips tightly around a spacer and slowly breathe in as you press down the inhaler (see Figure C). You don't have

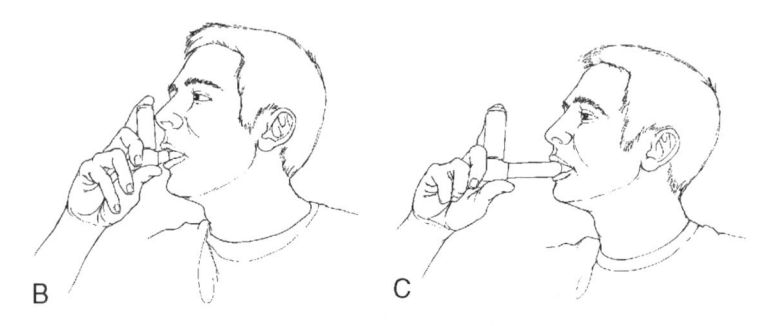

B C

to time everything perfectly because the spacer "holds" the medication until you inhale. It does the timing for you. If you sometimes end up coughing or gagging when you use an inhaler, a spacer can help.

There are different types of spacers. Ask your health care provider to explain how spacers work and suggest one to try. As with any inhaler, be sure to practice using an inhaler with a spacer while you're still in your doctor's office.

How Much Medicine Do You Have Left?

One tricky thing about inhalers can be figuring out how many "puffs" remain in the canister after you've used it a while. There is no perfect way to do this. Of course, if the canister is new, it's full, and the product label will tell you how many puffs of medicine it contains. You might try keeping track of how many times you use a new inhaler. You also can check (very roughly) your inhaler by placing it (not the mouthpiece!) in a cup of water. If the inhaler sinks to the bottom of the cup, it's full. If it bobs up and down, with the bottom end above the water, it's about half-full. Last, if the inhaler floats sideways in the water, resting on top, it's empty. Keep in mind, however, that this water test gives only a rough idea of how much medication you have left.

Cleaning Your Inhaler

It's important to keep your inhaler, mouthpiece, and spacer clean. Every day, you should rinse the inhaler and spacer with warm water and place them on a towel to dry. Twice a week, wash the plastic mouthpiece with warm water and a mild dishwashing soap. Let it air dry, too.

New-and-Improved Inhalers

People with asthma have been using MDIs for more than 40 years. During that time, the inhalers haven't changed much. But they are changing now. The drug companies that make inhalers are improving them.

Some of the changes are minor, such as remaking the mouthpiece to better fit your mouth, for example. Other changes are major. One new computerized device attaches to many inhalers and records the amount of medicine they contain. It also releases medication after you have begun inhaling, so you don't have to time things perfectly. In fact, several inhalers offer this kind of "breath-actuated" timing mechanism.

Using A Dry Powder Inhaler (DPI)

Some people aren't comfortable inhaling medication as a fine mist or spray. If you try an MDI and don't like it, you might consider using a dry powder inhaler (DPI). DPIs allow you to breathe in medication that is in a powder form. These inhalers are less common than MDIs, but they can be used to take various quick reliever or long-term controller medications. Like MDIs, most people over age 5 can use a DPI.

The DPI technique is different from the MDI technique. To use a DPI, you close your mouth tightly around the mouthpiece and inhale deeply and quickly. It's important not to exhale (breathe out) back into the inhaler—you will "lose" the medication. Ask your health care provider to explain how to use and clean a DPI. As with any inhaler, make sure you practice using it in your doctor's office and get written instructions.

Using A Nebulizer

No matter what the variety, every inhaler requires you to breathe in medicine, fairly quickly, from a small device. Some people find this difficult. In particular, children under age 5 and anyone with severe asthma might do better with a nebulizer rather than an MDI or PDI. A nebulizer works like an inhaler, only it's attached to a compressed air machine that helps you slowly, easily inhale asthma medication over about 10 minutes. You can take a variety of quick reliever and long-term controller medications with a nebulizer. The nebulizer has several parts: a cup to hold the medicine; a mask (usually for children under age 2) or a mouthpiece attached to a T-shaped part; and plastic tubing to connect this equipment to the compressed air machine.

Here's how to use a nebulizer correctly:

1. Wait one hour after eating before using your nebulizer. Alternatively, you can use the nebulizer before eating. Wash your hands before you get started.

2. Measure the amount of saline (salt water) solution and medicine to go into the nebulizer cup. Most people like to buy pre-mixed medication that you can just pour into the cup.

3. Attach the mouthpiece to the T-shaped part and then attach this to the nebulizer cup. (If you're using a mask instead of mouthpiece, fasten it to the cup.)

4. Put the mouthpiece in your mouth, and tightly close your lips around it. (Or place the mask on your face.)

5. Turn on the air compressor machine.

6. Slowly take deep breaths in through your mouth.

7. Hold each breath for a second or two before breathing out.

8. Repeat this procedure for about 10 minutes, or until all the medicine is gone from the cup.

Cleaning Your Nebulizer Daily

It's very important to clean your nebulizer every day. If bacteria builds up in your nebulizer, you can inhale it and get an infection. Keeping your nebulizer clean will also make it last longer. Ask your health care provider exactly how to clean the equipment. In general, you should clean your nebulizer every time you use it by doing the following:

1. Rinse the mask or mouthpiece and T-shaped part in warm water—sterile or distilled water is best—for about 30 seconds. (Do not wash the tubing.)
2. Put the pieces on a towel to air dry.
3. Put the mask or mouthpiece and T-shaped part, cup, and tubing back together. Connect the tubing to the compressed air machine, turn on the machine, and let it run for 10 to 20 seconds. This dries out the inside of the nebulizer.
4. Take the tubing off the compressed air machine. Store the nebulizer in a sealed plastic bag.
5. Cover the compressed air machine.

Cleaning Your Nebulizer Weekly (or Every Two Weeks)

In addition to daily cleaning, you should clean the nebulizer more thoroughly once or twice a week. To do this cleaning:

1. Wash the mask or mouthpiece and T-shaped part with a mild dishwashing soap and warm water. Rinse these pieces under warm water for 30 seconds.
2. Next, soak these pieces for 30 minutes in a solution that is one part distilled white vinegar and two parts distilled water. Afterward, pour out this solution. (Don't use it again.)
3. Again, rinse the nebulizer parts under warm running water for about a minute. Sterile or distilled water is best.
4. Let the pieces dry on a clean towel.
5. Put the pieces together, connect them to the tubing, and connect the tubing to the compressed air machine. Turn the machine on and let it run for 10 to 20 seconds.
6. Take the tubing off the compressed air machine. Store the nebulizer in a sealed plastic bag.

7. To clean the compressed air machine, rub it with a damp, slightly soapy cloth or sponge. Do not put too much water or soap on the machine, and never place the machine in a tub of water.

8. Cover the compressed air machine.

What To Remember About Inhaling Asthma Medicine:

You Have A Choice. When deciding how to inhale quick reliever or long-term controller medications, you have several options. MDIs are the most popular way to inhale asthma medicine. But you also can try a dry powder inhaler or, if you have severe asthma, a nebulizer. Consider using a spacer, which makes inhaling medication easier. Keep in mind that inhalers are improving. Ask your doctor about different types.

Technique Matters. Your inhaler only works if you use it correctly. Learning how takes time, patience, and practice. Ask your health care provider how to use an inhaler. While still at the doctors' office, practice. Also, get written instructions about using inhalers. Last, bring your inhaler to your check-up visits. Each time, show your doctor how you're using it. All this may sound like a lot of effort just to take your medication. But it's worth it. Good inhaler technique will help you get the full effect of your medication.

MANAGING YOUR MEDICATION OVER TIME

As you've learned, many doctors try a "step-down" approach to asthma treatment. You might start taking one level of asthma medicine and then, as your symptoms improve, gradually begin taking less and less medication. Eventually, you'll be taking the least amount of medicine needed to control your symptoms. Because asthma can quickly change—for better or worse—your health care provider will adjust your medicine plan carefully and slowly.

Here's an example: If you begin your medicine plan

by taking a moderate dose of daily corticosteroids, you might maintain this medicine level for several weeks. Then, if your symptoms are under control, your doctor may lower your dosage of corticosteroids by a fourth. You would then maintain *this* medicine level for some time, perhaps 2 to 3 months. If your asthma is still under control, you might cut back your medicine dosage again. And so on. In the end, most people with asthma benefit from taking some minimum level of daily medication.

Throughout this process, you and your doctor will work together to fine-tune your medicine plan. During regular follow-up visits, you'll review your medication, breathing ability, symptoms, and asthma triggers. Here is your chance to express concerns and ask questions. (I talk more about this in Chapter 5, "Managing Your Asthma Day to Day.") Eventually, you will learn how to gradually alter your medicine plan on your own. Don't try this at the beginning, however. Changing your medicine too suddenly can cause your symptoms to get much worse.

IS YOUR MEDICINE PLAN WORKING?

Before you can fine-tune your medicine plan, you must be able to evaluate it. You need to know when your medication works and when it doesn't. How can you tell? Remember that your goal is not to simply breathe a little better, part of the time. When your medicine plan is working, your breathing should be almost normal, no matter what time of day or what you're doing. A few questions can help you judge how well your medication works. Ask yourself:

- Is my medication causing side effects?
- Do I wake up at night, coughing or wheezing, more than twice a month?
- Have I recently missed school or work because of my asthma?
- If I try to be active—from running errands to running around the block—do I have a hard time breathing?

- Have I gone through more than one canister of inhaled beta$_2$ agonists this month? More than one canister over the past 2 months, even?
- During a recent asthma attack, did my inhaled quick reliever medication fail to work?
- Has my asthma sent me rushing to the hospital or doctor's office?

If you answered yes to any of these questions, reconsider your medicine plan. Perhaps your medication is not controlling your symptoms as well as it should. There are several possible reasons why. One common problem, as I mentioned, is inhaler technique. If you're not using your inhaler correctly, you may not be getting enough medication. Or maybe you've been sick, and your illness has aggravated your asthma. Perhaps you've moved, and you're much closer to an asthma-triggering allergen than before (for more on allergens and immunotherapy used to treat them, see Chapter 3, "Asthma-Proofing Your World"). Last, it might simply be the case that you're taking too little medicine to begin with.

No matter what the reason, tell your health care provider if you think your medication isn't working. Together, you can figure out how to fix the problem. If a respiratory infection is to blame or if a severe asthma episode has sent your symptoms spiraling, your doctor may suggest you try a short prescription of oral corticosteroids to get your asthma back under control. You might try a different kind of medication or just more of the kind you already have.

Remember: taking control of your asthma is an ongoing process. Use this chapter as a general guide to medication. Your health care provider will help you apply these principles to your personal asthma treatment. Then, you'll be making the most of your medication—and your health.

SUMMARY

- Medication is a critical part of your asthma treatment. There are two basic types of asthma medicine: quick

relievers and long-term controllers. The exact medications (and the amount) that's right for you depends on the severity of your asthma. Together, you and your doctor will create a medicine plan. Depending on your asthma symptoms, this plan will change over time.
- Most asthma medication is inhaled, rather than oral (liquid or pill form). Inhaled medication goes straight to your lungs and works quickly. You can breathe in medication using a metered dose inhaler, a dry powder inhaler, or a nebulizer. What works best depends on your comfort level and ability.
- For asthma medicine to work, you need to take it as prescribed, even if you feel fine. If you're inhaling medication, know the proper techniques for using an inhaler correctly. Using an inhaler correctly ensures that you are getting the full dose of medicine.
- Ask your doctor how often you should be taking any medication. If your symptoms do not improve, or if you need a lot of medicine to feel better, your medication isn't working as well as it should. There can be many reasons for this. If you think your medication isn't working well, tell your doctor. You may try new inhaler techniques, different medicine, or a different dosage.
- As in all of your asthma treatment, your health care provider is your partner. Asthma medication can be complicated. Ask questions. Express any concerns you may have. Whatever you do, don't simply start taking less, more, or no asthma medicine; your symptoms could get worse quickly. Instead, call your doctor. Together, you can adjust your medication to make you comfortable, confident, and in control of your health.

ACTION PLAN

You're now ready to take the next steps:
- Review your medicine plan. Ask yourself: Are my asthma symptoms under control? Does my medication seem to be working? Am I taking the prescribed amount?

- If you use an inhaler, check to be sure you're using it properly.
- Make a list of any questions or concerns to share with your doctor during your next check-up.
- Read Chapter 5, "Managing Your Asthma Day to Day," to learn more about controlling your asthma as time goes by. Medication is just one part of treatment. Eliminating asthma triggers and tracking your breathing ability also are important.

Chapter 5

Managing Your Asthma Day To Day

Asthma stays under control when you are in charge. That's why managing your asthma every day is essential, even when your breathing is fine. If you're concerned that asthma management will bog you down, don't worry. Monitoring your asthma will become a part of your daily routine—as easy as you find it now to brush your teeth, shower, eat, sleep, and do all your other everyday tasks.

Managing your asthma everyday has many benefits. You'll be able to prevent trips to the emergency room. You'll find that you won't have to think twice about what your asthma will and won't allow you to do. Daily asthma management will keep your airways at their best and let you be active without asthma symptoms. In this chapter, you'll learn how to use a personal written asthma management plan. You will also learn how to use a peak-flow meter and asthma diary to observe subtle changes in your airways that may lead to an asthma attack—even before wheezing and other symptoms become apparent to you. Your asthma management plan maps out what to do based on your peak-flow scores and changes in symptoms that you note. It's as if you are your own patient.

Such self-monitoring is important initially after you have been diagnosed as having asthma. Whether you should monitor your asthma daily on a long-term basis depends on several factors, such as the severity of your asthma and your ability to tell if your airways are narrowing. Be sure to ask your doctor whether he or she recommends long-term self-monitoring of your asthma.

PEAK-FLOW METERS AND YOUR PERSONAL BEST

You could guess whether your airways are narrowing based on your perceptions. But perceptions can be deceiving. A peak-flow meter will give you a more accurate idea of what's happening in your airways.

A peak-flow meter is a portable, low-priced device about the size of a softball. Easy to use, it measures how well air is moving through your airways. The rate at which your lungs do this is called your peak expiratory flow rate (PEFR). A peak-flow meter is meant to monitor, not diagnose asthma.

A peak-flow meter can tell you whether your airways are narrowing hours or days before you feel any asthma symptoms or any wheezing can be heard through a stethoscope. Knowing your PEFR, you can consult your asthma management plan, which is described in detail later in this chapter, and take additional medicine early, before symptoms worsen. Your peak-flow readings will also help you and your doctor determine whether your medicine plan is working, when you should increase or stop certain medications, and when to get emergency care. A peak-flow meter can also help you identify your personal asthma triggers if you take readings around suspected triggers.

Who should use a peak-flow meter? In general, routine usage of a peak-flow meter is recommended for people who take asthma medications daily. However, in the first two to three weeks after your asthma diagnosis, you may use a peak-flow meter to evaluate your airways' response to maintenance medications, pinpoint any relationship over time between changes in your readings (as many as four or more times a day) and your exposure to asthma triggers (for more about asthma triggers, see Chapter 3, "Asthma-Proofing Your World"), and establish your personal best peak-flow reading. Finding your personal best is detailed later in this section.

Your health care provider will let you know if you need to use a peak-flow meter for long-term monitoring. According to the guidelines published in 1997 by the National Heart, Lung and Blood Institute, you will need to use a peak-flow meter daily on a long-term basis if you are at least 5 years of age and have moderate or severe asthma. Basically, there are three basic levels of asthma: mild, moderate, and severe.

If you have *mild* asthma, you get brief attacks just once or twice a week. Your asthma symptoms will be intermittent. Your breathing, as measured by a peak-flow meter, is about 80 percent as strong as it should be. Your breathing ability is about the same during day and night. If this description fits you, your health care provider will probably suggest you inhale a short-acting beta$_2$ agonist during your asthma attacks. This quick-reliever medication should help you breathe easier in a matter of minutes. You may also need to keep track of your daily breathing patterns by using a peak-flow meter at home. (For more information about your medication plan, see Chapter 4, Asthma Medications.)

If you have *moderate* asthma, you often get asthma attacks more than twice a week. Your attacks may involve more serious coughing, wheezing, and breathing problems. Your breathing ability, as measured by peak-flow rate, is 60 to 80 percent of what's normal. You have a harder time breathing at night. If this description fits you, your health care provider may recommend taking an inhaled corticosteroid (a long-term controller) every day and a short-acting beta$_2$ agonist (a quick reliever) during asthma attacks. You'll need to use a peak-flow meter at home to learn how much your breathing improves with this medication.

If you have *severe* asthma, you have an asthma attack almost every day. You may also have a chronic cough. You wake up at night because you can't breathe well. Your breathing ability, as measured by a peak-flow meter, may be about half of what it should be. If this description fits you, your doctor may suggest using a higher dosage of an inhaled corticosteroid (a long-term controller) every day and a short-acting beta$_2$ agonist (a quick reliever) during asthma attacks. Again, you'll want to use a peak-flow meter at home to track your breathing ability.

How and When To Use a Peak-flow Meter

Your health care provider should show you how to use a peak-flow meter. Because correct usage is essential to monitoring your asthma, your doctor will ask you to show him or her how you use it during follow-up appointments.

To ensure consistent readings, you should use the same peak-flow meter or, at least, the same brand, over time. Whenever you buy a new peak-flow meter, you should reestablish your personal best with the new one. You should also clean your peak-flow meter regularly to get accurate readings. Follow the cleaning instructions provided with your device. Finally, be sure to bring your peak-flow meter to follow-up visits with your doctor.

To use a peak-flow meter, you do not need to wear a nose clip. Follow these steps:

1. Move the indicator to the bottom of the numbered scale.
2. Stand up.
3. Take a deep breath, filling your lungs completely.
4. Place the mouthpiece in your mouth. Close your lips around it. Do not put your tongue inside the hole.
5. Blow out as hard and fast as you can in a single blow.

Write down the number on the meter. However, if you coughed or made a mistake during the above five steps, don't record that number. Do it over again. Then, repeat steps 1 through 5 two more times, and write down your best peak-flow reading of the three blows in your asthma diary. This is your PEFR.

Figuring Out Your Personal Best

Now you're on your way to finding your personal best. A personal best peak-flow number is the highest PEFR you can achieve over two to three weeks when your asthma is controlled well. In other words, you feel good and do not have any asthma symptoms. The so-called "normal" peak-flow readings are based on height, sex, and weight. However, this number is based on averages. Best peak-flow readings may differ from person to person, which is why it's important to find your own, *personal* best.

To find your personal best, you will track your PEFR two to four times a day during those initial two to three weeks. You will take readings when you wake up but before taking medications and between noon and 2 p. m. If you take short-acting inhaled beta$_2$ agonists for quick relief, you will also take peak-flow readings before and after you take this medicine. Your health care provider may recommend additional times for you to take readings.

The personal best is then used to shape your asthma management plan. You should have your personal best reassessed periodically to check the progress of your asthma. In children with moderate to severe asthma, this two- to three-week monitoring period to determine a personal best should be repeated every year. Peak-flow readings generally increase as a child grows.

A peak-flow meter can also help you find your triggers. To use the peak-flow meter to find out whether a suspected trigger is a true trigger, first take a peak-flow reading before you are exposed to a suspected trigger. Then, take a second reading following exposure. Your doctor can help you use your peak-flow meter for this purpose.

GREEN, YELLOW, AND RED: YOUR PERSONAL ASTHMA MANAGEMENT PLAN

Based on your personal best peak-flow number and your medication plan, your doctor will write down your personal asthma management plan similar to the one below. The asthma management plan uses the color scheme of a traffic light, telling you what medicines to take based on that day's peak-flow reading.

These color zones help you make the decisions your doctor wants you to make when he or she is not there.

You have been entrusted to call the shots in your asthma care. For asthma control to be at its best, bear in mind that you and your doctor work as a team. Be sure to tell him or her your observations and recordings from your peak-flow monitoring and other aspects of your asthma self-care. This valuable information will help the two of you further refine your asthma management plan shown below.

Green means GO: Your GREEN ZONE is _____, 80 to 100 percent of your personal best. Breathing is good with no cough, wheeze or chest tightness during work, school, exercise or play.

ACTION:
- Use preventive (anti-inflammatory) medicine as directed in your daily treatment plan.

Yellow means CAUTION: Your YELLOW ZONE is _____, 50 to less than 80 percent of your personal best. Asthma symptoms are present (cough, wheeze and chest tightness). Your peak-flow number drops below _____, or you notice:

- increased need for inhaled quick-relief medicine
- increased asthma symptoms when you wake up in the morning
- waking up at night with asthma symptoms

ACTION:
- Take ____ puffs of your quick-relief (bronchodilator) medicine.
- Take ____ puffs of your anti-inflammatory medicine _____ times/day.
- Begin/increase treatment with oral steroids:
  Take ____mg of _____ at _____AM _____PM.
- Call your doctor at (____)____-_____ or emergency room (____)____-_____.

Red means STOP: Your RED ZONE is _____, 50

percent or less of your best. DANGER! Your peak-flow number drops below _____, or you continue to worsen after increasing treatment according to the directions above.

ACTION:
- Take _____ puffs of your quick-relief (bronchodilator) medicine. Repeat ____ times.
- Begin/increase treatment with oral steroids. Take _____ mg now.
- Call your doctor now at (_____)_____-_____. If you cannot reach your doctor, go directly to the emergency room (_____)_____-_____. (List here other important phone numbers including nearby relatives or friends and taxi service: _____

At any time, call your doctor if:

- asthma symptoms worsen while taking oral steroids
- inhaled bronchodilator treatments are not lasting four hours
- your peak-flow number remains or falls below _____ even though you are following your asthma treatment plan.

WRITE IT DOWN: YOUR ASTHMA DIARY

You'll chart your progress in an asthma diary, an essential tool for monitoring your asthma. An asthma diary is easy to set up. You can buy any inexpensive notebook or three-ring binder at an office supply store. The advantage of using a binder is that you can make photocopies of blank copies of your weekly charts instead of redrawing them each time you need one.

The diary will help you become familiar with subtleties of your asthma symptoms. If you notice that your asthma is worsening, then you should call your doctor sooner rather than later when you are at greater risk of a severe asthma attack. I have found that many people with asthma wait until it's too late. Minor symptoms are much easier to control than a severe asthma attack.

In fact, any doctor, including myself, wants you to seek help when asthma symptoms are in their early stages instead of waiting for things to become critical. If you are concerned about your airway status, then call your doctor. Let him or her know what your peak-flow readings have been and your symptoms. You'll have this information because you've recorded it in your asthma diary. At the very least, you can get some feedback—and feel reassured. Don't think of the phone call as an inconvenience to your doctor.

Here's a rough outline of what your asthma diary should look like (your health care provider may have sample asthma diaries for you to use). Here's an explanation of some of the elements of the asthma diary.

1. Each page in your asthma diary covers one week.

2. You should fill in the blanks next to "My predicted peak flow," "My personal best peak flow," "My green (OK) Zone (80 to 100 percent of personal best)," "My yellow (Caution) zone (50 to 80 percent of personal best)," and "My red (Danger) zone (below 50 percent of personal best, according to your asthma management plan that you and your doctor have designed."

USING YOUR ASTHMA DIARY

1. Take your peak-flow readings every morning (A. M.) when you wake up before you take any medications and every night (P.M.) at bedtime. Try to take your readings at the same time everyday. Write down the highest reading of three tries in the row marked "Peak-flow reading" in the space below date and time.

2. Is your peak-flow reading in the green, yellow, or red zone? Depending on which it is, follow your asthma management plan accordingly.

Weekly Asthma Diary

___ My predicted peak flow
___ My personal best peak flow
___ My Green (OK) Zone (80–100% of personal best)
___ My Yellow (Caution) Zone (50–80% of personal best)
___ My Red (Danger) Zone (below 50% of personal best)

Date	a.m.	p.m.	a.m.	p.m.	a.m.	p.m.	a.m.	p.m.	a.m.	p.m.	a.m.	p.m.	a.m.	p.m.
Peak-flow reading														
No asthma symptoms														
Mild asthma symptoms														
Moderate asthma														
Serious asthma symptoms														
Medicine used to stop														
Urgent visit to the doctor														

3. In the space below that day's peak-flow reading, put an "X" in the box that matches the symptoms you have when you take a peak-flow reading. No symptoms means no wheezing, coughing, chest tightness or shortness of breath even with normal activity. Mild symptoms means symptoms during physical activity, but not at rest and that you can still sleep and be active. Moderate symptoms occur while at rest and may keep you from sleeping and being active. Serious symptoms occur at rest (although wheezing may not be present) and you may have difficulty walking or talking. In addition, muscles in neck or between ribs pull in when breathing.

4. Mark an "X" in the box in the row for medicine use if you took extra asthma medicine to stop your symptoms.

5. If you had to go to your doctor's office, emergency room, or hospital for treatment of an asthma attack, write an "X" in the row labeled "urgent visit." Notify your doctor by the next business day that you went to an emergency room or hospital for treatment.

DEALING WITH ASTHMA ATTACKS

Up to this point, I've focused on controlling your asthma day to day. By now you know that everyday management of asthma—noticing warning signs and acting on them—will greatly decrease your chances of having an asthma attack. Nevertheless, you and your health care provider should develop a written action plan for managing asthma attacks just in case.

The first thing you should always be alert to is warning signs. Remember, asthma attacks rarely occur without physical changes in your body happening hours before symptoms appear. These warning signs are different for everyone. Actually, you may have different warning signs from one time to the next. To get to know your warning signs, recall your last asthma attack and see if you had any of the warning signs listed below. Mark the ones that are your warning signs and write in additional ones, if you had any. Be sure to tell your doctor and family what your warning signs are. Finally, number from one to three what your most common warning signs of an asthma attack are.

- Drop in PEFR
- Chronic cough, especially at night
- Difficulty breathing
- Chest begins to get tight or to hurt
- Breathing faster than normal
- Getting out of breath easily
- Tired
- Itchy, watery, or glassy eyes
- Itchy, scratchy, or sore throat
- Stroking chin or throat
- Sneezing
- Head stopped up
- Headache
- Fever
- Restlessness
- Runny nose
- Change in face color
- Dark circles under eyes

Knowing these warning signs means that you can begin treatment early. Make sure you take the correct amount of medicine at the times your doctor instructed. If your asthma management plan includes increasing dosage or adding a second medicine, take them as prescribed. CALL YOUR DOCTOR before taking more medicine than he or she recommended. Then, take these steps:

- Remove yourself from the trigger, if you know what it is, to improve your response to medication.
- Remain calm. Ask family members, coworkers and others with you to stay relaxed as well. Examples of ways to stay calm include talking to someone, watching TV, listening to music, or using relaxation/breathing techniques, such as repeating to yourself in a quiet room, "I can stay calm."
- Rest.

- Note changes in body signs, such as wheezing, coughing, trouble breathing, and posture. If you have your peak-flow meter with you, measure your peak-flow five to ten minutes after each treatment to see if your peak flow is getting better.
- Be sure to know when to seek emergency medical care immediately. Review the list below regularly. Get emergency care when:

  - Your wheeze, cough or shortness of breath worsen, even after you have taken your medicine and given it time to work (about 5 to 10 minutes for most inhaled bronchodilators). Your doctor can tell you how long the medications he or she has prescribed take to work.
  - Your PEFR goes down, does not improve after you use a bronchodilator, or drops to 50 percent or less of your personal best.
  - Your breathing gets difficult and your chest and neck are pulled or sucked in with each breath. You are hunching over. You are struggling to breathe.
  - You have trouble talking or walking.
  - You stop playing or working and cannot start again.
  - Your lips or fingernails appear gray or blue. If this happens, GO TO THE NEAREST EMERGENCY ROOM NOW!

Because an asthma attack can occur away from home, you should be sure to keep information, including information on seeking emergency care and important phone numbers, with you at all times. If you need help, don't hesitate to call a family member, friend, or neighbor if needed. When treatment is not working or you are concerned, call your doctor's office, a clinic, or hospital for help.

During an asthma attack, you should not drink a lot of water. Your normal amount of water is fine. Although tempting, do not breathe warm, moist air from the shower or a humidifier. In addition, do not breathe into a paper bag held over your nose. Also, don't take over-the-counter cold medications without consulting a doctor.

SUMMARY

- Asthma stays in control when you are in charge. Daily asthma management will keep your airways at their best and keep you free from asthma symptoms.
- A written personal asthma management plan, a peak-flow meter, an asthma diary to track your symptoms and peak-flow readings, and an action plan for dealing with asthma attacks are key tools for daily control of your asthma. Your health care provider should show you the correct way to use a peak-flow meter, a device that will tell you what's really happening in your airways.
- You will find your personal best using a peak-flow meter. Your personal best and your medicine plan will shape your asthma management plan. Depending on the severity of your asthma, you may take peak-flow readings daily for long-term asthma management. You should have your personal best reassessed periodically.
- You and your health care provider should put together an action plan for dealing with asthma attacks. You should know what the common warning signs of an asthma attacks are as well as your own warning signs.

How will it feel to be in charge of your asthma? I think you'll find that being in control makes you feel good emotionally and physically. You will be like an athlete who knows his or her body well, including its potential and limits. I have found that knowing what's going to happen is far better than not knowing, which is why I think you will see the benefits of keeping an asthma diary. Of course, your asthma diary can track other important information relating to your asthma care, so use it as much as possible. For example, you can tape your asthma goals to the inside cover. Perhaps, you may want to track your medications and keep phone numbers of your doctor all in one place. It's also instructive to read through it occasionally to see your progress.

ACTION PLAN

With all of that you have learned in this chapter, you are ready to:

- Start an asthma diary. Buy a notebook and make up several weeks' worth of charts. Keep the notebook near your bedside along with your peak-flow meter.
- Review the warning signs of an asthma attack and what to do. Explain the warning signs and what to do with friends, coworkers, and family. Post important phone numbers (doctor, hospital, emergency room, taxi service, and ambulance service) in your asthma diary and near phones. Carry these numbers with you at all times.
- Make a list of questions and concerns about your asthma management plan, asthma diary, peak-flow meter, and action plan for dealing with asthma attack before your next appointment. Discuss your asthma management plan with your doctor. Ask him or her for help when you are having trouble controlling your asthma or using your peak-flow meter.
- Select which of the next four "Living With Asthma" chapters apply to you and read them.

Chapter 6

Living With Asthma: Special Types of Asthma

For some people with asthma, the symptoms of asthma only appear at certain times. In these special types of asthma, it may be easy to pinpoint the cause. For example, if you only get asthma symptoms when running, you may have exercise-induced asthma. Some people have "cough-variant" asthma, in which the only symptom is coughing. They may even be surprised that this annoying cough is indeed asthma. Some people only get asthma during certain seasons of the year—seasonal asthma—because of airborne allergens, such as pollens and molds. Another special kind of asthma is occupational asthma, triggered by inhaling irritants at work.

If you experience only special types of asthma, read this chapter. In it, I discuss the special types of asthma and management plans for them. This chapter is also helpful if you suspect that your asthma occurs only at certain times.

I also urge you to speak with your health care provider. Together, you can identify the cause and manage your asthma. Your doctor also may be able to help you deal with concerns unique to special types of asthma. What do you tell your boss? Should you stop exercising? Can you stay on the varsity team?

EXERCISE-INDUCED ASTHMA

What do track star Jackie Joyner Kersee and diver Greg Louganis have in common? Both have won Olympic medals. Both also have asthma. They and other athletes—including "weekend warriors"—know that it's possible to exercise even if you have asthma. Most people with asthma get symptoms during vigorous activity.

For some, exercise is the only trigger. Either way, you don't have to stop being active, but you do need to take special care. If your asthma only occurs during a game of tennis, pick-up basketball, a run through the park, or other sports activity, you have exercise-induced asthma. Having this form of asthma doesn't mean you have to avoid these sports. Often, using an inhaled bronchodilator before, during, or after your workout (or sometimes all three) can control this kind of asthma.

Trigger

Exercise-induced asthma—sometimes called exercise-induced bronchospasm—is believed to be caused by a loss of heat, water, or both from your lungs because you are breathing more heavily than normal. Typically, the air you inhale is cooler and drier than air in your lungs, which is warm and moist. The exchange of air leaves your airways dry and cold. There is disagreement, however, whether cold or dry air is the true culprit.

During exercise-induced asthma, your airways constrict minutes after you become active. You may cough, wheeze, feel tightness or pain in your chest, or get other asthma symptoms. Exercise-induced asthma usually happens during or minutes after vigorous activity, peaking about 5 to 10 minutes after you stop. Symptoms go away 20 to 30 minutes later.

Diagnosis

Before you decide for yourself that your asthma occurs only during vigorous activity, see your doctor. Sometimes, you may have asthma symptoms aside from exercise, but you don't realize it. To diagnose exercise-induced asthma, your doctor will take a medical history and give you an exercise challenge test. During this test, you will ride a stationary bicycle or run/walk on a treadmill. Your doctor will measure your airway capacity before, during, and 20 minutes after your test. Your doctor also may ask you to monitor your asthma using a peak-flow meter for two weeks while not exercising. (See Chapter 5, "Managing Your Asthma Day to Day," for more on peak-flow meters.) This monitoring period will determine if you have asthma symptoms away from exercise. A peak-flow meter can tell you when your airways are narrowing.

Medicine Plan

The goal of a medicine plan for this kind of asthma is to help you maintain normal activity levels without asthma symptoms. Your health care provider will tell you how to prepare your airways for exercise or other strenuous activity. As with other forms of asthma, the key is to treat your airways before symptoms begin—or at least worsen.

For most people with exercise-induced asthma, inhaling a short-acting $beta_2$ agonist within an hour before exercise prevents asthma symptoms. You can usually count on the medication working for about two to three hours. Other medications your doctor may prescribe are cromolyn and nedocromil. Again, these medications are taken before exercise.

You also may get less—and less severe—exercise-induced asthma if you use anti-inflammatory medications on a regular basis. You and your doctor will decide if this option is better for you. Both types of medications are described in more detail in Chapter 4, "Asthma Medications."

Management Plan

Before you start a sports game or other heavy activity, take time to stretch and warm up. Warm-ups and stretching are essential to prevent muscle injury. But you may also find that by warming-up you may not have to take additional medication during exercise. Also, you may find that gradually improving your overall fitness may lessen the severity of your asthma symptoms, too.

Should you avoid certain sports and other activities? That depends on the severity of your symptoms and how well you can control them. Avoid working out if you have a viral infection, such as a cold; if the temperature is very low; or if pollen and pollution are high. If you are exercising in cold weather, cover your mouth and nose so that you inhale warm, moist air.

If you consistently find that running sparks asthma despite your efforts to control your symptoms, you may have to switch activities. Some cold weather sports can trigger symptoms, too, such as ice hockey and cross-country skiing. So do nonstop activities, like basketball, soccer, field hockey, and long-distance running. However, staying in shape and following your asthma medication plan closely may allow you to participate in whatever sport you like—and even to compete.

Examples of less strenuous sports you might choose are:

- light jogging
- walking
- biking
- hiking
- swimming

Activities with short bursts of vigorous activity are also good choices, including:

- short-distance track and field events
- football
- wrestling
- golfing
- surfing
- gymnastics
- baseball

Be sure to tell coaches or teachers if you have exercise-induced asthma. If your child has exercise-induced asthma, talk to his or her coaches, teachers, camp counselors, and relevant others. (For more on children and asthma, see Chapter 9, "Living With Asthma: Through The Years.") They should know that your (or your child's) participation in sports is fine, and that you will use an inhaled medication for activity. Your health care provider can give you a letter stating that you can participate in sports and may require inhaled medication before, during, and after the activity. If you are in competitive sports, such as the Olympics, you may need to notify the governing board for that sport or competition that you use asthma medication. The U.S. Olympic Committee has set standards for drug use during competition. If you have questions or concerns, you may contact their Drug Control Hotline at 1-800-233-0393.

COUGH-VARIANT ASTHMA

Cough-variant asthma is common, especially in children. If you have cough-variant asthma, your main symptom is coughing, frequently at night. During the day, you feel fine and have no other symptoms. In fact, you may even find it hard to believe that your cough is asthma because you don't wheeze or have other typical asthma symptoms.

If you find you're not sleeping at night because you keep waking up coughing, you may have cough-variant asthma. Or, if you find that you are coughing during the day but do not have a cold or other illness, you may have cough-variant asthma. Your doctor may ask you to monitor your asthma using a peak-flow meter for two weeks. The goal of this monitoring period is to see how your breathing ability changes over time. A peak-flow meter can tell you whether your airways are narrowed.

Once your diagnosis is established, you and your health care provider will develop a personal asthma management plan for you, as discussed in Chapter 5, "Managing Your Asthma Day to Day." This plan includes asthma medications and a medicine plan, described in Chapter 4, "Asthma Medications."

SEASONAL ASTHMA

If you have seasonal asthma—that is, asthma that occurs only in seasons of the year when certain pollens and molds are highest in your area—read Chapter 3, "Asthma-Proofing Your World" and Chapter 5. In these chapters, you'll find information on dealing with seasonal allergens. You and your doctor will decide what medications you should take before and throughout the season in which your asthma appears. For more information about medications, read Chapter 4.

OCCUPATIONAL ASTHMA

Sometimes, your workplace can cause asthma. About 2 percent of all cases of asthma are related to the job. What are the clues? Symptoms usually appear within a few months to about four years after your first exposure. Your coworkers might have similar symptoms, such as wheezing, chest tightness, and difficulty breathing. You should suspect occupational asthma if you notice that asthma symptoms go away when you're away from work for several days, such as for a vacation or at the end of a weekend.

You might miss this cause-and-effect relationship if your symptoms appear only after you've been at work for several hours. Asthma symptoms may occur within your first hour at work—or as much as eight hours later, or even at night.

Triggers

Some 250 agents may cause occupational asthma. These agents are present in both manufacturing plants and offices. Widely used in many industries, including automobile, airplane, train, and steel manufacturing, toluene isocyanates are responsible for most cases of occupational asthma. This type of chemical is used in spray painting; insulation installation; and in the making of plastics, rubber, and foam. Isocyanate-induced asthma affects nearly 10 percent of workers exposed to this chemical.

Other common triggers include dander from laboratory animals, dyes, formaldehyde, persulfate, chloramine-

T, anydrides, amines, proteolytic enzymes (used in detergents), cotton dust, gum acacia (a chemical used in color printing), and wood dust. Exposure to plant products (for example, green coffee beans, papain and castor beans), hydrochloric acid, ammonia, or sulfur dioxide also can trigger asthma. Other potential irritants are cold, heat, dust, and humidity in the workplace.

Veterinarians and other animal workers may also develop asthma as a result of exposure to dander from animals. Health care workers may get asthma symptoms from the aerosolized proteins found in latex gloves or when combining powdered medications. Workers in places where flour is used in great amounts may get so-called baker's asthma. Metal workers, carpenters, adhesive handlers, forest workers, seafood processors, hairdressers, cleaning staff, bakers, electronics workers, carpet makers, and pharmaceutical workers are among the many professionals who are at higher risk for occupational asthma because of known asthma triggers in the workplace.

One way to identify the potential asthma triggers in your workplace is to ask for Material Data Safety Sheets. By law, these sheets must be made available to all workers. Your personnel office should have these sheets on file. They list the chemicals and substances used in your particular workplace. However, the sheets may not contain all the substances that may trigger your asthma.

Diagnosis

Because asking about the potential health effects of your work environment can be a delicate issue, it's best to get a careful asthma diagnosis. You and your health care provider need to determine that your asthma symptoms occur only at work—and are not just asthma symptoms that are worsening as a result of allergens or irritants from outside the workplace. Also, your doctor needs to rule out bronchitis or an asthma-like condition called reactive airway dysfunction syndrome, which is the result of strong exposures to gases, dust, or fumes.

First, your doctor will want a detailed description

of your work history and workplace. You should try, if possible, to tell him or her all substances used at your workplace, whether you work with them or not. However, some substances may cause delayed asthma symptoms. So even if you don't get symptoms while you're working with a particular substance, it might still be a cause.

You and your health care provider also should work together to document any work-related changes in airflow through your airways. You will need to monitor your asthma for two to three weeks and keep accurate records of your peak-flow reading. You will record when symptoms and exposures occur and when you use a bronchodilator. You'll also measure and record peak-flow readings every two hours while awake. Your health care provider also may suggest other tests and/or refer you for further evaluation for confirmation. Specific challenge tests, during which you are exposed to the suspected trigger, may be available.

Management Plan

Once you have documented that your asthma is related to a workplace trigger, you can work with onsite health care providers or managers. The Americans with Disabilities Act requires that employers make every effort toward "reasonable accommodation" by improving the workplace for employees with occupational asthma. You can talk about whether avoidance, ventilation, or use of respiratory protection will help. For example, you might need to use a special type of filtering mask or a smoke-free environment at work.

Another option is changing jobs within your company to avoid exposure to the irritant, if it is known. Ask your doctor to contact the American Thoracic Society, which publishes guidelines for the evaluation of impairment and disability in people with asthma. Your doctor should also contact the appropriate public health agency for further assistance.

If you return to the same job, you should have close medical follow-up. However, if your asthma worsens, you may eventually need to change jobs or even professions. The medications prescribed for occupational asthma are the same as for other types of asthma (See Chapter 4). Even after you leave your job, you may still need to take medication for several months.

SUMMARY

- Some people with asthma only get asthma symptoms at certain times or during certain situations. The common kinds of asthma are exercise-induced asthma, cough-variant asthma, seasonal asthma, and occupational asthma.
- Exercise-induced asthma occurs whenever a person exercises or engages in other heavy activity. You need to get a proper diagnosis to see if your asthma symptoms appear only during exercise. Sometimes, you may have asthma symptoms away from exercise, but you don't notice them. You can continue your exercise program and do other vigorous activities with a proper asthma management plan. The key is to treat your asthma before you work out.
- In cough-variant asthma, the main symptom is coughing, often at night. Your doctor may ask you to monitor your asthma using a peak-flow meter for a two-week period when you are not exercising. This monitoring period will uncover whether you have other asthma symptoms at other times. Once your diagnosis is made, you and your health care provider will tailor an asthma management plan for you.
- Seasonal asthma is asthma that appears only in certain seasons of the year, when pollens and molds are highest in your area. You and your doctor will decide what medications you need to take before and during that particular season in which your asthma appears.
- Occupational asthma accounts for about 2 percent of all cases of asthma. You should suspect that your asthma is job-related if your symptoms disappear whenever you are away from work for several days. You and your health care provider need to confirm that your asthma symptoms occur only at work and are not simply

getting worse at work. You and your health care provider should also work together to document that you are showing work-related changes in airflow through your airways. Avoiding triggers, better air ventilation, and use of respiratory protection may help.

If you suspect that your asthma is a "special type," then this chapter should help you pinpoint the cause of your asthma. Your self-awareness will help you link your symptoms to a certain time of year, the activity you were doing, or, perhaps, your workplace. Fortunately, for each special type of asthma, solutions are available that will help you maintain a healthy and normal activity level.

ACTION PLAN

With the information you have read about in this chapter, you are now ready to:

- Talk to your health care provider about the special types of asthma that you've learned about. Prepare a list of questions and concerns before your next office visit if you want more information or need clarification.
- Learn proper warm-up exercises to do before you workout or participate in other strenuous activities. Check in your local library or bookstores for books that can show you how.
- Ask your doctor whether you should take any allergy medications—prescription or over-the-counter—if you have seasonal allergies.
- Continue to monitor your asthma, no matter which type you have. Check with your doctor if you are unsure about using your peak-flow meter correctly or taking medication properly. If you find that you are increasing your medications, talk to your doctor—the sooner, the better.
- Report any changes in your asthma—for better or worse—to your health care provider.
- Reread the relevant chapters in this book, if you have questions on medications, triggers, or asthma management.

Chapter 7

Living With Asthma: Pregnancy

When you're pregnant, asthma takes on new meaning. You are breathing for two. Asthma not only affects you, but it also could affect your unborn baby. That's why it's so important to treat your asthma carefully during pregnancy. The basic rules of asthma management—avoiding triggers, taking medication, and monitoring your breathing—still apply. But each rule carries some special considerations.

As you read this chapter, you'll learn how asthma changes during pregnancy; how to avoid asthma triggers; which medications are safe and unsafe; how asthma affects each trimester of pregnancy, labor, and delivery; what to do during an asthma attack; and how to handle special pregnancy situations.

As always, you have help in controlling your asthma. Depending on the situation, you may work with an obstetrician, a nurse-midwife, or an asthma specialist. In each instance, the message is the same: you need to—and you can—stay in control of your asthma while pregnant.

We are still learning how asthma and pregnancy interact. Our major source of information is the 1993 "Report of the Working Group on Asthma and Pregnancy," sponsored by the National Asthma Education Program. The working group was made up of a dozen doctors in different specialties, all of whom had treated pregnant women with asthma. Their report has become the major guideline for doctors everywhere.

ASTHMA DURING PREGNANCY

How Does Asthma Affect You?

Let's start by talking about how asthma affects you directly. As you learned in earlier chapters, different people have different asthma symptoms. This holds true for mothers-to-be, too. Your asthma may be mild, moderate, or severe. *Mild asthma* causes only an occasional asthma attack, with few symptoms in between. If you have *moderate asthma,* you often get attacks more than twice a week, and you have a harder time breathing. *Severe asthma* causes an asthma attack almost every day and a chronic cough or difficulty breathing. The severity of your asthma determines how much medication, monitoring, and trigger avoidance you need to do.

Asthma is hard to predict. If you've had asthma during an earlier pregnancy, you might have a similar experience (in symptoms, medication, etc.) this time around. On the other hand, some women who've never had asthma develop it for the first time while pregnant. Meanwhile, about a third of women with asthma get worse during pregnancy. Why? Researchers aren't sure. They do know, however, that several common conditions during pregnancy can aggravate asthma, including upper respiratory infections, sinus infections, colds, and gastroesophageal reflux, which causes heartburn.

Most asthma-related pregnancy problems begin when asthma goes uncontrolled. If you're not breathing well and your lungs are inflamed, you're more likely to develop other problems. One of the most important is high blood pressure, which can lead to a condition called preeclampsia. Preeclampsia is characterized by high blood pressure and swelling during pregnancy, which, if not recognized, can lead to a serious condition called ecampsia, which causes seizures. You can develop health complications even if you don't notice your asthma symptoms are slowly getting worse.

Keep in mind, however, that for many women, asthma doesn't change during pregnancy. You might even be surprised to find that your asthma symptoms actually improve. Again, researchers aren't sure why this happens. Hormonal changes during pregnancy might help keep the body's asthma-causing chemicals in check.

The bottom line is that your asthma could stay the same, improve, or worsen during your pregnancy. All this variation means that it's important to stay on top of your asthma. Together, you and your health care provider can quickly notice any changes in your breathing and respond with medication or increased monitoring.

How Does Asthma Affect Your Baby?

The other person asthma affects is your baby. To develop normally, a fetus needs a steady supply of oxygen from its mother's bloodstream. But uncontrolled asthma can decrease the amount of oxygen in your blood. When that happens, your baby may not get enough. A baby who receives too little oxygen could be born sicker, smaller, or even earlier than normal.

ASTHMA TREATMENT GOALS

The good news is that you can avoid these problems. As with asthma during any time of life, proper treatment can help you—and your baby—stay healthy. With your asthma under control, you usually can expect:

- Fewer asthma symptoms, such as hard breathing, even at night
- No limits on moderate exercise or other activity appropriate during pregnancy
- Normal or near-normal tests of lung function
- Few or no asthma attacks
- No trips to the emergency room or hospital for asthma
- Easy use of medication with few side effects for you or your baby
- Delivery of a healthy baby

The key to achieving these goals is to create a personal

asthma management plan for your pregnancy. Your obstetrician or nurse-midwife can help you understand how asthma can change during pregnancy. Your primary care provider can also help. Feel free to ask questions, gather information, and voice concerns. If you have severe asthma or allergic asthma, you also should see an asthma specialist during your pregnancy.

When you're pregnant, you need to consider carefully the three features of asthma management: triggers, medication, and monitoring.

AVOIDING ASTHMA TRIGGERS

As you learned in Chapter 3, "Asthma-Proofing Your World," many people get asthma attacks when they come in contact with certain "triggers," or substances to which they are sensitive. These triggers can also increase your airways' sensitivity, leaving your lungs inflamed and more prone to asthma attacks in the future. Again, inflammation happens over time, quietly, so you may not even realize your asthma is slowly getting worse.

There are two basic types of asthma triggers: allergic and nonallergic. Most asthma triggers fall into the first category. When you have allergic asthma, your body overreacts to certain substances with a predictable inflammatory response. The most potent allergen triggers come from the dander, saliva, and droppings of pets; house-dust mites; and cockroaches. Other allergens include molds and pollen. Nonallergen triggers can be strong odors (paint or perfume, for example), outdoor air pollutants, and tobacco smoke.

Why do triggers matter? If you can avoid the triggers that aggravate your asthma, you can stay healthy with the least amount of medicine possible. And when you're pregnant, that's a good idea. Asthma medications—when taken at the right time, dosage, and type—are safe during pregnancy. Still, it's wise to limit the amount of medication you and your baby receive in order to prevent side effects.

Asthma triggers are different for different people.

Working with your doctor, you'll learn which triggers affect you the most. Chapter 3 reviews major asthma triggers in detail and shows you how to avoid them. Here are just a few steps to take while you're pregnant. Depending on your asthma, some, but not all, of these tips will apply:

- Don't smoke—and don't sit near anyone who is.

    Not only is cigarette smoke a potent asthma trigger, but it also decreases your lung function. And the chemicals in tobacco smoke can cross the placenta, affecting your baby's lungs, too. Every pregnant woman should avoid smokers and smoking.
- Consider removing pets from your home.

    We all love our pets. But if you're allergic to animal allergens (like pet dander), then your dog, cat—and even birds or mice—may make your asthma worse. Even if you remove the pet from your house, its dander can linger for several months. A 3% tannic acid spray can help clean out remaining allergens. At the very least, keep pets out of your bedroom and keep the bedroom door closed at all times. If you plan to keep your pet, washing it once a week may help. If your friends have pets, ask your doctor about taking asthma medicine before visiting their homes.
- Protect yourself from house-dust mites.

    These mites give off an allergen that can spark asthma problems. The house-dust mite allergen makes its way into bed mattresses, covers, pillows, carpets, upholstered furniture, clothes, and soft toys. If you are allergic to this allergen, you should take steps to avoid it, as outlined in Chapter 3.
- Avoid other allergens.

    Mold and cockroach allergens can both cause asthma attacks in some people. Keeping your house clean and dry (with a dehumidifier) may make allergens less likely to build up in the home. You can avoid some outdoor allergens, like pollen, by staying inside during the afternoons in warm summer months. Keeping windows shut and air conditioning on also may help.

Some people with allergic asthma find relief in immunotherapy, in which you receive a small amount of an allergen (in a shot) until your body gradually gets used to that allergen. If you're pregnant and already receiving 'allergy shots,' your doctor may tell you to continue. Side effects are rare. Occasionally, however, a person getting allergy shots has a bad reaction, called anaphylaxis. To prevent anaphylaxis, your doctor may suggest you do not begin immunotherapy for the first time while pregnant. After your baby is born, you can try allergy shots.

ASTHMA MEDICATIONS

To learn about asthma medications in general, read Chapter 4, "Asthma Medications." Much of the information is the same whether you're pregnant or not. However, when you're pregnant and asthmatic, there are four medication rules to remember:

1. Asthma Medicine Is Safe. Many women get nervous about taking medication while pregnant. However, research has shown that it's much safer to take asthma medication than it it is to let your asthma go untreated. If you take the right medication (and the right amount), your asthma will improve with little risk to you or your baby.

2. Inhaled Medication Is Best. Asthma medications that you inhale as a spray or mist usually are safer than oral (pill or liquid) varieties. When you inhale a drug, it goes directly to your lungs. When you swallow a drug, it travels in your bloodstream throughout your body. You—and your unborn baby—are more likely to experience side effects when this happens. Along the same lines, it's good to use a spacer with your asthma medicine inhaler (see Chapter 4). This device helps deliver most of the medicine to your lungs, and you end up swallowing less.

3. Use Medicine With A Safe History. Ask your doctor which asthma medications have a safe history of use in pregnant women. Over time, some drugs have been used repeatedly, while newer ones do not have the benefit of past experience. Also, check with your doctor about the proper dosage of medication. The right amount depends on your weight at the time you take the drug.

4. Learn About Asthma Medications. The more you know, the more confident you'll feel. No drug is absolutely without risk. However, asthma drugs are generally safe.

Which Drugs Are Safest For Pregnant Women?

The Working Group on Asthma and Pregnancy has reviewed all the existing studies on asthma medicine in pregnant woman and offers the following information. Remember: before you take any medication during pregnancy, talk to your doctor. Together, you will decide the medicine that's right for you.

Quick Relievers

The most common quick relievers are short-acting beta$_2$ agonists. These drugs include albuterol (brand names: Proventil®, Ventolin®), pirbuterol acetate (Maxair®), terbutaline sulfate (Brethaire®), bitolterol mesylate (Tornalate®), and metaproterenol sulfate (Alupent®, Metrapel®). When inhaled, short-acting beta$_2$ agonists can stop an ongoing asthma attack, usually within 5 to 10 minutes.

Because these medications are used only as needed, you should not be taking them more than several times a week. At this level, the drugs do not appear to harm pregnant women or their unborn babies. Most research on these drugs, however, has involved women using the medication late in pregnancy. In some cases, the drugs can lead to tremors or hypoglycemia (low blood sugar) in newborns. These conditions can be treated and reversed.

An alternative drug is theophylline (Theo-Dur®, Respbid®, Slo-Bid®, Theo-24®, Theolair®, Uniphy® l, Slo-Phyllin®), which is released in your body over a period of hours. Theophylline does not work during an acute asthma attack. However, some people who normally wake up wheezing during the night find that taking theophylline before bedtime helps. It has been used extensively in pregnant women, and it does not appear to cause harmful side effects at normal doses.

Long-Term Controllers

In general, inhaled corticosteroids, or anti-inflammatory medications, do not appear to cause side effects in the mother or fetus. Inhaled medicine is best. There are at least three drug compounds available as inhaled asthma medication: beclomethasone (Beclovent®, Vanceril®), dexamethasone sodium phosphate (Decadron Phosphate Respihaler®), triamcinolone acetonide (Azmacort®), and flunisolide (AeroBid®, AeroBid-M®).

Among inhaled corticosteroids, beclomethasone is the one pregnant women have used most. For that reason, many doctors prefer to prescribe it over the others. It's possible that this drug might enter your bloodstream, but researchers believe it's unlikely that harmful amounts would reach your baby. By comparison, there's little information about the effects of dexamethasone, triamcinolone, and flunisolide on pregnant women.

Oral (also called systemic) corticosteroids are sometimes used to help you get your asthma quickly under control. For pregnant women, these drugs are less safe than the inhaled variety. High doses of oral corticosteroids may lead to a baby that's smaller than normal. In one study, women who took 10 milligrams of prednisone (Deltasone®, Liquid Pred®, Metocorten®, Orasone®, Panasol®, Prednicen-M®, Sterapred®) throughout pregnancy had a slightly increased risk for low-birth weight babies.

Two common alternatives to corticosteroids are cromolyn sodium and nedocromil sodium. These drugs often are used before exercise to prevent exercise-induced asthma. They also might help ease asthma symptoms caused by inhaling cold air or sulfur dioxide. In pregnant women, cromolyn sodium appears safe. However, we have little information about nedocromil sodium.

In recent years, several new types of long-term controller medications have become available. We are still collecting information about their use during pregnancy. These drugs include long-acting $beta_2$ agonists (Salmeterol®) and leukotriene modifiers like zafirlukast (Accolate®) and zileuton (Zyflo®).

In review, the Working Group recommends these asthma drugs for pregnant women:

- Quick relievers: inhaled $beta_2$ agonists, theophylline
- Long-term controllers: cromolyn sodium, beclomethasone, prednisone

Other recommended drugs include:

- Antihistamines: chlorpheniramine, tripelennamine
- Decongestants: pseudophedrine, oxymetazoline
- For cough: guaifenesin, dextromethorhpan
- Antibiotics: amoxicillin

Which Drugs Are Unsafe For Pregnant Women?

There are a few drugs you should avoid taking while pregnant, if possible. Ask your doctor about specific medications if you have a condition that requires medicine. In general, avoid taking:

- Decongestants: These over-the-counter medicines are used to treat colds.
- Live virus vaccines: Ask your doctor before getting any vaccine while pregnant. Killed-virus vaccines, in which the virus is deactivated entirely, are okay.

- Immunotherapy: These allergy shots are okay if you already are taking them. If you aren't, wait until after your pregnancy to begin.
- Iodides
- Over-the-counter inhalers: Don't use over-the-counter medications, like epinephrine, phenylephrine, or brompheniramine. Instead, ask your health care provider which medicine is right for you.

Medication and Breast-Feeding: A Special Note

Many women with asthma prefer to breast-feed their babies. You can do this safely. It's true that nearly all medications enter breast milk, but the amount of medicine usually is low. It's rare that a baby is affected. The American Academy of Pediatrics has reported that a range of asthma drugs are safe for mothers of nursing infants, including terbutaline, a quick reliever, and prednisone, a long-term controller. One drug, theophylline, may cause vomiting or shakiness in sensitive newborns. As with drugs during pregnancy, it's a good idea to ask your doctor which asthma medications have a history of safe use during breast-feeding.

MANAGING ASTHMA THROUGH PREGNANCY, LABOR, AND DELIVERY

If you have asthma, one of the most important things you can do while pregnant is monitor your breathing. Asthma can change from month to month, getting better or worse. If you keep track of your breathing ability, you'll know when your asthma is beginning to change. Right away, you'll know to call your doctor, alter your medication level, or prepare for a coming asthma attack. When you act quickly, you can prevent yourself and your baby from getting too little oxygen. Similarly, fetal monitoring is important. Your doctor will help you monitor your baby's health, making sure the baby is safe as your pregnancy develops.

Each trimester of pregnancy—as well as labor and delivery—brings its own asthma monitoring options. The types of monitoring depend on how well your asthma is under control and how well your baby is growing. In general, here's what you can expect:

First Trimester: Months 1–3

Monitoring Your Health

Some women develop asthma for the first time during pregnancy. If that's true for you, your first step is a diagnosis. To diagnose asthma, your doctor will run a series of lung function tests. These tests are described in detail in Chapter 2," Working With Your Health Care Provider."

Diagnosing asthma during pregnancy can be tricky because pregnant women often experience shortness of breath, or dyspnea. When you're pregnant, rising hormone levels, weight gain, and other physical changes can affect the rate at which your lungs and heart work. Using objective breathing tests, like spirometry, will help your doctor determine if asthma really is the cause of your breathing difficulties.

If you've already been diagnosed with asthma, you'll need to get and record what's called a "personal peak-flow best." A peak-flow meter is a device that measures how well your lungs use and exhale air. The rate at which your lungs do this is called your peak expiratory flow rate (PEFR). Peak-flow meters are discussed in Chapter 5, "Managing Your Asthma Day To Day."

Your doctor will show you how to use a peak-flow meter at home. Every day for a couple of weeks, you will record your PEFR. Using your records, your doctor will help you determine your personal peak-flow best—this is the best job your lungs can do. Your personal best becomes a baseline, or point of comparison. Then, as you measure your PEFRs throughout pregnancy, you can see when your breathing changes. If you have moderate or severe asthma, your doctor will suggest you take a peak-flow reading every day. If your PEFRs drop, your asthma may be getting out of control.

It's important to monitor your breathing because it can change without you noticing. Even with few symptoms, you may be taking in less oxygen, which endangers your baby. Peak-flow readings will alert you as soon as your breathing changes.

When it comes to acute asthma attacks, these episodes appear to peak between 24 and 36 weeks of pregnancy. Below, you'll learn what to do during an asthma attack.

Monitoring Your Baby's Health

Much like you, your baby benefits from getting an initial assessment, or "baseline" measurement, between 12 to 20 weeks of pregnancy. This time, the measurement is fetal growth rate. Using a sonogram, your obstetrician or nurse-midwife will measure your baby's size. A sonogram is an easy, painless procedure in which a health care provider applies sound waves (ultrasound) to your abdomen. (Although "ultrasound" refers to the type of sound waves used, and "sonogram" refers to the actual procedure, the two terms are sometimes used interchangebly). The projected images of the baby—which help show its size and location—can be watched and recorded on a video screen. With these initial sonogram measurements, health care providers can be sure your baby is growing at a healthy rate in later months.

If everything seems normal, your health care provider will simply measure the size of your abdomen from 20 to 32 weeks of pregnancy. During this time, the height (in centimeters) of your unborn baby equals his or her age in weeks. In other words, a fetus will grow at an expected rate. If the readings indicate your baby is not as big as expected, your doctor will perform another sonogram to double-check.

Second Trimester: Months 4–6

Monitoring Your Health

As your pregnancy progresses, think "maintenance." By now, you have forged a partnership with your health care provider and are taking asthma medication. You also know how to avoid asthma triggers and measure your daily peak-flow readings.

During this time, it's also important to be on the lookout for other conditions that might aggravate your asthma. If you get a chest cold, for example, your asthma could quickly get worse. Upper respiratory infections are the most common cause of asthma exacerbations in pregnant women.

One of the best things you can do now is communicate with your health care provider. If you have questions or concerns, express them. Feel free to make a list of questions and call your health care provider. When you get the answers you need, you'll feel confident about your health.

Monitoring Your Baby's Health

Again, if everything seems normal, your doctor will measure your abdomen at regular check-ups, keeping track of the measurements to ensure that your baby is growing at a normal rate. If you have severe asthma, or if your asthma has gotten out of control, your baby's health may be monitored with periodic sonograms, which provide a more precise picture of fetal growth.

Third Trimester: Months 6–9

Monitoring Your Health

As you approach your due date, it's time to start planning for your delivery. Talk to your doctor about what will happen if you get an asthma attack during labor, for example. Although asthma attacks during labor are rare, you'll feel confident if you know what to expect. According to studies, the last four weeks of pregnancy (weeks 36–40) often are the most symptom-free for women with asthma.

Monitoring Your Baby's Health

During your last trimester, your health care provider will pay close attention to your growing baby, making sure he or she seems to be growing well. If your asthma is under control, you may only need weekly check-ups. At home, you'll also do daily "kick counts," in which you count the number of times you feel the baby kick during, say, 10 minutes. Kick counts help asses the baby's activity level.

If you have severe asthma, or if your baby seems to be growing more slowly than normal, your doctor also may do sonograms or electronic fetal heart rate monitoring. In this last procedure, health care providers lightly place a belt—much like seat belt—around your abdomen. This belt is attached to a machine that records your baby's heartbeat. The recordings let health care providers make sure your baby's heartbeat is normal.

If you have a serious asthma attack that might affect your baby's oxygen level, your doctor may do what's called "intensive fetal monitoring." Intensive fetal monitoring refers to one or several types of monitoring, such as the electronic fetal heart rate tests mentioned above. Health care providers will continue this kind of monitoring until they're sure everything is okay.

Labor and Delivery

If you have been controlling your asthma throughout your pregnancy, you're in good shape for labor and delivery. It's rare that controlled asthma causes any problems while your baby is being born. Your doctor probably will suggest you continue using your (regularly-scheduled) asthma medication at this time.

As a precaution, your peak-flow rate, or PEFR, will be taken when you're first admitted to the hospital. PEFR measurements will be taken every 12 hours afterward, as long as your labor continues. If needed, your health care provider may give you oxygen to breathe.

Another precaution is fetal monitoring. If your asthma is mild and under control, health care providers will ask you to undergo 20 minutes of electronic fetal heart rate monitoring. This is routine. If the monitoring results are normal, you may need further monitoring at timed intervals. On the other hand, if you have severe or uncontrolled asthma, your doctor may suggest continuous, or intensive, fetal heart rate monitoring.

During labor and delivery, health care providers will be careful to choose drugs that do not cause an asthma attack. For example, if your doctor needs to induce labor, oxytocin is the drug of choice. For pain relief, an epidural analgesic is safe. If you need a general anesthetic, your health care provider will likely choose ketamine. If you experience vaginal bleeding, or postpartum hemorrhage, after childbirth, you probably will be given oxytocin again.

There are a few special situations that require extra care. Preterm labor is the major one. If you have an asthma attack late in pregnancy, you may experience uterine contractions. These contractions do not usually progress to labor. Occasionally, however, they do. If you are taking an oral (systemic) beta$_2$ agonist, you may be given magnesium sulfate to calm the contractions.

WHAT TO DO DURING AN ASTHMA ATTACK

If you have an asthma attack at any time during your pregnancy, you need to act quickly to get your breathing back under control. If your breathing does not improve soon, you may take in too little oxygen, which could harm your baby.

The secret to quick action is an asthma management plan. Together, you and your doctor will write down what to do before, during, and after an asthma attack. Chapter 5 explains such a plan. It's important for you to have a plan you're comfortable with. In general, your asthma management strategy will help you:

- Recognize the warning signs of an asthma attack. Daily peak-flow readings can signal an asthma attack before it even occurs. This kind of early warning system will give you time to react by calling your doctor. You may need to increase your medication at this point.
- Use inhaled beta$_2$ agonists properly to regulate breathing during an attack.
- Know what to do if an asthma attack is severe. It's important to call your doctor or go to the emergency room if your asthma does not respond to medication. Also, call your doctor if your baby's "kick counts" decrease following an asthma attack. At your doctor's office or the hospital, health care providers might give you medication or oxygen, monitor your breathing, and monitor your baby's heartbeat. Their goal is get your breathing under control and make sure you and your baby are fine.
- Know what to expect following an attack. Recovery may take a few days, and you may need medication throughout this time. Ask your doctor what medicine to take and for how long.
- Remember what NOT to do during an asthma attack. Don't rely on over-the-counter drugs like antihistamines or general inhalers. Also, don't try to cure yourself by drinking lots of liquids or breathing warm, wet air, like in a shower.

SPECIAL PREGNANCY SITUATIONS

Every woman is different, and every pregnancy presents its own challenges. Maybe you have an existing health condition other than asthma, for example. Or perhaps you feel nervous or scared about being pregnant and having asthma. Rest assured that you're not alone. Pregnancy is wonderful, but it can be trying. Here are a few special situations that could affect you:

Anxiety

When you're pregnant, you're faced with change. Bringing a baby into the world brings countless questions. Will you have a boy or a girl? Will your baby be healthy? Are you ready to be a parent? Adding asthma to the list of uncertainties can add more stress. Now is the time to ask for emotional support. Ask your friends or family members to help. Also, your doctor can answer questions and recommend a pregnancy discussion group. Last, look over Chapter 11, "For More Information," for a list of organizations that offer support groups or information on asthma.

Diabetes

If you have insulin-dependent or gestational diabetes, your asthma medication could make your diabetes worse. Oral, or systemic, beta$_2$ agonists and corticosteroids may affect your blood sugar level and increase your insulin requirements. In order to find the right combination of medicine, you'll need to work closely with the doctors treating your diabetes, asthma, and pregnancy.

Sinusitis or Rhinitis

These conditions cause a runny nose, stuffy head, or other cold symptoms. Normally, they're not a problem. Occasionally, however, sinusitis or rhinitis can aggravate asthma. Tell your doctor if you are bothered by cold-like symptoms that won't seem to go away. Depending on the cause, you can take medication to find relief.

SUMMARY

- When you become pregnant, you're no longer the only one affected by asthma. If untreated, your asthma could

decrease the amount of oxygen your baby gets in the womb. A decreased amount of oxygen could cause your baby to be born sicker, smaller, or even earlier than normal. Similarly, asthma can lead to other conditions—like high blood pressure—for you, too.
- Fortunately, you can control your asthma during pregnancy. Asthma is different for different people, and the right treatment depends on your own condition. You may have mild, moderate, or severe asthma. Throughout pregnancy, your asthma can change. But your treatment plan follows the same principles. As at any time in life, asthma management relies on three things: avoiding asthma triggers, taking the right medication, and monitoring your (and your baby's) breathing.
- When you're pregnant, avoiding asthma triggers becomes very important. In doing so, you minimize the amount of medication you need.
- Medication is a vital part of controlling your asthma. Several varieties of quick-reliever and long-term controller medications have been deemed safe in pregnant and breast-feeding women. It's much safer for you and your baby to take medication than to let your asthma spiral out of control.
- In each stage of your pregnancy, your health care provider will monitor your health and your baby's health.
- Throughout your pregnancy, you need to act quickly before or during an asthma attack. When you create a personal asthma management plan, you'll learn what to do. Keep this written plan, and use it as a guide.
- Each pregnancy brings its own challenges. You may have a health condition, such as diabetes, that can affect (or be affected by) your asthma. Working with your health care providers, you can keep all your conditions under control.

ACTION PLAN

No matter how far along you are in your pregnancy, you can take a few steps to review your health and plan for the future. Now that you've read this chapter, you're ready to:

- Review your peak-flow readings and be sure your asthma is under control
- Rethink your medication plan and avoidance of triggers if you're having asthma symptoms
- Reread the relevant chapters in this book if you have questions about medicine, triggers, or monitoring
- Talk to your doctor about what to do during an asthma attack and what to expect during labor and delivery. Make sure your written asthma management plan is easy to find and use.
- Continue measuring your baby's "kick counts" and report any changes to your health care provider
- Report any changes in your asthma—for better or worse—to your doctor

Chapter 8

Living With Asthma: Everyday Situations

Let's say you've met your goals for asthma management. You are leading an active life with few or no asthma symptoms. With the guidance of this book and your health care provider, you've learned how to control your asthma—every day, in fact.

This chapter takes you one step further in your asthma management plan. It discusses typical situations, such as having a cold or taking a vacation, that crop up now and then. Everyone faces these situations. However, you will need to give them special attention because they may affect your asthma and your management plan. Knowing what to do ahead of time will cause less of a disturbance in your asthma management plan—and, consequently, your daily activities. You'll learn what to do when you have an illness, including some tips on avoiding the common cold and flu; when you need surgery; when you experience stress; and when you are planning a trip and are traveling. I also suggest questions that you can ask your health care provider in each situation.

UNDER THE WEATHER?

It's morning and you don't quite feel well. Should you go to work or school or stay home? In general, you can probably go to the office or school if you have a stuffy nose but are not wheezing or if have a little wheezing that goes away after taking your asthma medicine. It's probably a wise decision to stay home from work if you have:

- a sore throat; swollen, painful neck glands; or other physical signs of infection

- a temperature greater than 100° Fahrenheit (F) [oral] or 101° F (rectal)
- wheezing or coughing that still bothers you after 1 hour after taking your asthma medicines
- weakness or fatigue that makes it difficult to perform your daily activities
- difficulty breathing or breathing very fast
- peak-flow reading below 65 to 70 percent of your personal best and no response to treatment

If you are unsure whether you should stay home, call your doctor. Be prepared to describe your symptoms and when they appeared.

The Common Cold

You know the hallmark symptoms of the common cold: runny nose, sore throat, and body aches. Colds are caused by a virus that infects the respiratory system. Over 200 different viruses have been identified that cause the common cold. A cold can trigger asthma symptoms because it further irritates your airways, sinuses, nose, throat, and lungs. Although there is no cure for the common cold, you still can keep it manageable.

How to Manage It

Before you get a cold, ask your doctor ahead of time what you can do to manage the symptoms of the cold and how you should adapt your asthma management plan. Colds last about 7 to 10 days, whether or not you take over-the-counter medications. Your doctor will not prescribe antibiotics because these drugs treat bacterial infections only. You may find that you have to increase your asthma medications because your cold is triggering asthma symptoms. Before taking over-the-counter cold medications, consult your health care provider. He can advise you about which medicines to avoid because they may interact adversely with your asthma medications.

Which Cold Medicine is Best?

The rule of thumb is that less medication is better. In general, you should only take cold medications that treat the symptoms you have rather than taking broad medication that treats all possible symptoms. As with any over-the-counter medication, be sure to read the directions, list of ingredients, and the warnings on the label. Store medications safely out of the reach of children. For a stuffy nose, ask your doctor about using saline nose drops rather than decongestant nose drops, which can be habit-forming. For aches, take acetaminophen. (For more information on aspirin sensitivity in people with asthma and aspirin substitutes, see Chapter 3, "Asthma-Proofing Your World.")

Prevention

We get colds more often in winter than at other times of the year—not because of the cooler temperatures but because of changes in the way we live during cold climates. We heat our homes, which decreases humidity. As a result, our usually moist sinus passages become drier. Moist sinuses protect us from cold viruses and other foreign invaders. In winter, we also stay indoors more, which means that we increase our contact with others. Greater interaction raises our chances of coming into contact with any of the viruses that cause the cold.

Cold germs are spread through touching or breathing in cold germs. You can adopt a few simple habits to avoid catching a cold:

- Avoid shaking hands with a person who has a cold.
- Wash your hands often, especially when you interact with a person who has a cold.
- Avoid touching door knobs, telephones, or other objects a person with a cold may have just touched. Wipe them first.
- Cover your nose and mouth whenever you sneeze or cough. Members of your household should do the same.

- Keep your hands away from your nose, mouth, and eyes.
- Use disposable tissue to blow your nose. Throw out the tissue immediately after each use.
- Don't drink beverages from the same glass, eat from the same plate, or use the same utensils of someone who has a cold.

Influenza (Flu)

Commonly called the flu, influenza is an infection of your airways that is caused by three main types of viruses: A, B and C. The flu usually strikes in winter. At first, you feel weak and you may have a headache and muscle aches. As the flu progresses, you may get a sore throat, cough, and sniffles. The flu caused by the type C influenza virus is milder, and its symptoms are similar to those of the common cold. The flu spreads from person to person in the air. You can get the flu if you breathe in the droplets of an infected person that become airborne when he or she sneezes or coughs.

How to Manage It

Before flu season arrives, ask your doctor ahead of time what you can do to manage the symptoms of the flu and how you should adapt your asthma management plan. Like the common cold, the flu has no cure. Within the first 24 hours of experiencing flu symptoms, you should call your doctor. In people with lung or heart disease, he or she may prescribe amantadine, an antiviral medication. Amantadine may lessen the severity of your symptoms if you take it within 24 hours of the beginning of your symptoms. Otherwise, you should stay in bed until your fever goes away and take nonaspirin painkillers (See Chapter 3, "Asthma-Proofing Your World," for more information on aspirin sensitivity in people with asthma and aspirin substitutes) for relief of your aches. After you no longer feel weak, you may slowly return to your daily activities.

Prevention

Getting a flu vaccination is important for people who have respiratory diseases, such as asthma. Each fall, you should see your health care provider to get a flu vaccine. Your doctor may recommend that members of your household also get flu shots. Unlike other vaccines, such as those for smallpox and measles, the flu vaccine is good for only that winter's flu season for two reasons. First, the strain of flu virus differs from year to year, and your vaccination will only protect you from that particular strain. Second, the protection you get only lasts long enough to get you through the flu season.

The flu vaccine is only about 60 to 70 percent effective. Therefore, you still have a chance of getting the flu. Nevertheless, it is your best hedge against this illness. You should also follow the precautions for preventing transmission of the cold viruses that are outlined above, as the flu is spread similarly.

Sinusitis

Your sinuses are air-filled pockets located in the bones just under your nose. Mucus drains from the sinuses into your nose. When you have sinusitis, the lining of the facial sinuses swell because of a bacterial or viral infection. The infection is carried from the nose to the sinuses. Usually, sinusitis occurs after a cold. Sometimes, the infection results from a tooth abscess, severe facial injury, or contaminated water that travels up the nose when a swimmer leaps into water feet first without holding his or her nose.

When you have sinusitis, you may feel fullness or aches on either side of your nose or above your eyes, where the sinuses are located. You may also have a fever, a stuffy nose, a lack of a sense of smell and, sometimes, a nasal discharge due to the collection of pus in your sinuses.

How to Manage It

If you are prone to sinus infections, talk to your doctor before you get another one. Together, you can decide how you might adjust your asthma medications and treat your sinus infection. When you get a sinus infection, see your doctor. Your doctor will ask about your signs and symptoms, and you may have your sinuses x-rayed.

Some sinus infections are caused by viruses, and some are caused by bacteria. Antibiotics are prescribed for bacterial sinus infections but are useless against viral infections. However, it's difficult to tell initially whether a sinus infection is caused by bacteria or a virus. The test that's normally used to differentiate between the two types of infections—a culture—is very painful to perform on the sinuses, and so it's not used that often. Your doctor, then, may advise you to wait a week or two to see if your symptoms clear up spontaneously. If they do, your infection is probably viral. If they don't, your infection is probably bacterial, and you will need antibiotics.

One more note about antibiotics. It's important to take them as prescribed and to finish all the medication. If you don't follow your doctor's directions to the letter, the bacteria may persist and can cause serious problems.

Prevention

You may be able to prevent sinus infections by preventing colds. Follow the cold-prevention steps as described above. You should also avoid swimming in contaminated water. The local public health department may be able to tell you whether a lake or other body of water is safe for swimming.

Frequent Heartburn

The burning in your chest called heartburn is caused by the backflow of stomach acid into your esophagus. This backflow is called acid reflux. If you have chronic heartburn, you may have gastroesophageal reflux disease (GERD). GERD is common among people who have asthma and, in fact, occurs at a greater rate than among those in the general population. Coughing, choking, or wheezing during the night may also mean that you experience GERD during sleep. GERD may trigger asthma symptoms, and asthma symptoms and its management may worsen GERD.

Many studies have found a relationship between bronchospasms and acid reflux. However, researchers think that this relationship may be just one of several influencing factors that explain the higher rate of GERD among people with asthma. Another factor is theophylline usage, which is known to increase stomach acid. However, you should not stop taking any of your asthma medications without talking to your health care provider first.

How to Manage It

If you have frequent heartburn or poor control of your asthma symptoms at night, see your health care provider. He or she may you have a few tests to determine the cause of your heartburn and whether GERD is a problem. Your doctor may prescribe medications that suppress acid production and that prevent acid reflux. Several acid-suppressing medications are now available over the counter. However, do not take these medications without first seeking the advice of your health care provider.

Prevention

There are several steps you can take to prevent heartburn:

- Avoid eating or drinking 3 hours before going to bed.
- Raise the head of your bed on 6- to 8-inch blocks.
- Eat smaller meals at a relaxed pace.
- Maintain a healthy weight that is appropriate for your age, sex, and height. Being overweight places pressure on your esophagus.
- Do not lie down after eating.

PREPARING FOR SURGERY

Whether you are about to have elective or nonelective surgery, you will need to take special precautions since you have asthma.

Before surgery, you will receive a presurgical examination. During this examination, you will have the opportunity to ask questions and talk to the anesthesiologist. Before this examination, write down any questions and concerns that you have. Bring this list with you to the exam as well as your asthma diary and a list of all medications that you take, both over-the-counter and prescription. During the visit, review with your surgeon and your anesthesiologist the following: your asthma symptoms, medication use (especially if you have taken oral corticosteroids for longer than 2 weeks in the past 6 months) and your peak-flow readings.

Here is a list of questions you may want to ask your health care provider during the presurgical examination:

- Should I get a second opinion?
- What the risks and benefits of this procedure?
- What does the operation entail?
- Why do I need surgery?
- What are the nonsurgical alternatives, if any?
- What type of anesthesia will I receive?
- What will the recovery period be like?
- When can I go home? Do I need to stay at the hospital? If so, for how long?

You should also contact your health insurance company to check whether you need preauthorization for surgery and hospitalization.

STRESS AND ASTHMA

Your first home. A traffic jam. A job promotion. A death in the family. A vacation on the Mediterranean. A divorce. Some situations in your life can cause stress. No one leads a life free from stress. How do stress and other psychological factors affect a person with asthma? Researchers don't have the complete picture yet. Evidence thus far suggests that stress plays an important role in worsening asthma symptoms and may possibly be a risk factor for the increase in the prevalence of asthma. Although the evidence that stress can adversely affect asthma is as yet incomplete, it's still a good idea for you to decrease the stress in your life. Because you'll feel more relaxed, you may be better equipeed to follow your asthma management plan.

Stress management is a popular endeavor right now. Classes for stress management are offered at the local YMCA, adult education centers, hospitals, and American Heart Association. Your workplace may also offer these classes. Your health care provider or local hospital may know of stress management seminars in your area. You might sign up for a class or, if you prefer, read a book about stress management to learn specific relaxation techniques, such as deep breathing, progressive muscle relaxation, and meditation.

Here are some other stress management strategies that you might try:

- Decrease your load. Find things on your "To Do" list that really don't need to be done today, tomorrow, or ever. Learn to say "no."
- Get a good night's rest every night.
- Eat a balanced diet and don't eat on the run.
- Avoid caffeinated beverages and medications.
- Start an exercise program—gradually—and stick with it. (See Chapter 6, "Living with Asthma: Special Types" for information about exercise and asthma.) Yoga and walking are good choices.
- Take time for yourself. Read, play, go for walks, meet a friend for lunch.
- Take frequent breaks.
- Talk to a friend or loved one. Talking helps diminish your fears and concerns.

GLOBE TROTTING

Heading to a cottage on the beach or a resort on an exotic island? Whether you're going for a week in Nantucket or Tahiti, a little planning will help you keep your asthma under control while you are away from it all. Of course, if your asthma is not under control at home, be sure to fine-tune your asthma management plan before you go. For your trip, you will want to know all about the area that you're visiting, such as its climate, altitude, and humidity. Additionally, you will want to think ahead about the possibility of asthma triggers, your medication refills, and the location of doctors and hospitals.

You may want to select your location and time of travel based on your asthma triggers. For example, if mold is a problem for you, you may not want to go to a humid climate. When you pick out your vacation spot, talk to your health care provider and/or allergist. If you are traveling outside the United States, he or she can tell you what, if any, vaccinations you need to get. You will also want to learn about pollen and spore seasons in the region that you will visit.

The National Allergy Bureau (1-800-9-POLLEN), which is managed by the American Academy of Allergy, Asthma and Immunology, can provide you with information about pollen and spore seasons in the United States and around the world. Their information is based on average conditions. However, keep in mind that local weather can change and your sensitivity to airborne allergens can also influence the severity your symptoms. If you have any questions, ask your health care provider.

Here are additional tips for ensuring a pleasurable and memorable trip:

- Get a letter from your health care provider that summarizes your medical history, your asthma management plan, and medications. Keep this letter with you at all times.
- Ask your health care provider if he or she knows of a doctor who practices where you are vacationing. You will want to have the name of a doctor and a good hospital in the event of a medical emergency—especially if you are traveling in a foreign country. Having this information before you go is better than searching for medical care in an emergency. If your doctor doesn't know of anyone, contact a specialty organization's physician referral line. One such line is operated by the American Academy of Allergy, Asthma and Immunology (1-800-822-2762). See Chapter 11, "For More Information," for a listing of additional resources.

- Ask your health care provider whether he or she recommends that you wear a bracelet or carry a card that identifies you as a person with asthma.
- Ask your health care provider whether your medication schedule is affected if there is a time zone difference.
- Refill your medications so that you have enough for your whole vacation. You may want to get a second inhaler in case you lose one while traveling. If you belong to a managed care organization, contact member services and ask if they have a vacation refill program. Keep medications in their original containers. (Even when you are not traveling, you should never store medications in anything but their original bottles.)
- Pack medications someplace where you can get to them quickly during an emergency. Because losing your luggage is possible, place your medications in carry-on luggage.
- Keep a list of your medications—including the generic and brand name—along with dosages in your wallet or purse.
- Find out whether the hotel you are staying at has air conditioning and nonsmoking rooms.

SUMMARY

- You should stay home from work or school because of illness. In general, you can go to the office or school if you have a stuffy nose but are not wheezing or if have a little wheezing that goes away after taking your asthma medications. Stay at home if you have signs of a physical infection, such as a fever or sore throat; peak-flow reading below 65 to 70 percent of your personal best or no response to treatment; or weakness or fatigue. If you are unsure, call your doctor.
- The common cold, which is caused by a virus that infects the respiratory system, can trigger asthma symptoms. There is no cure for the common cold. We get colds more often in winter than at other times of the year because we stay indoors more. This change in

lifestyle means that we increase our contact with others. Cold germs are spread through touching or breathing in cold-causing viruses.
- Antibiotics treat only bacterial infections. They do not rid you of the common cold, the flu, or sinus infections that are caused by viruses.
- Frequent heartburn is due to the backflow of stomach acid to the esophagus. Gastroesophageal reflux disease (GERD), for which frequent heartburn is a symptom, is common among people who have asthma. Asthma symptoms that occur at night may be a sign of GERD. There are several medications available to control GERD.
- Before surgery, you need a presurgical exam. During this visit, you will need tell your surgeon and anesthesiologist about your asthma symptoms, medications you take and peak-flow readings.
- Stress may play a role in worsening asthma symptoms and may be a risk factor for the increasing incidence of asthma. However, more studies need to be done to understand the role stress plays in asthma. Nonetheless, even people who do not have asthma will benefit from learning stress management techniques, such as deep breathing, progressive muscle relaxation, and meditation.
- Travel may mean heading to a place where the asthma triggers are different from where you live. You may want to select a location and time of travel based on your asthma triggers. The National Allergy Bureau (1-800-9-POLLEN) can provide you with information about pollen and spore seasons in the United States and around the world. If your asthma is not well-controlled at home, your asthma symptoms will disrupt your travel, too.

This chapter has shown you how to adapt your asthma management plan and what to consider about controlling your asthma in special situations. Most situations simply require that you work with your health care provider ahead of time and put together an asthma management plan for these situations. By planning ahead, you can avert any disruptions in controlling your asthma. You can expect that your asthma will remain under control during these times when you are sick, stressed, or on vacation. In addition, you are now aware of problems or concerns that people with asthma run into more often, such as gastroesophageal reflux disease (GERD), and know that the problem is shared by other people with asthma. Plus, you can take steps to manage these problems.

ACTION PLAN

With the information you have read about in this chapter, you are now ready to:

- Start practicing cold and flu prevention strategies. For example, wash your hands often.
- Ask your doctor ahead of time about adjusting your asthma management plan when you have a cold or other illness.
- Talk to your doctor about which over-the-counter medications you may take. Take medications that treat only the cold symptoms you have. Avoid medications that contain aspirin.
- Make an appointment early in the fall for your yearly flu vaccination. You might want to mark your calendar to remind you to call in October for an appointment. Encourage household members to get flu shots as well.
- Use antibiotics properly and take them only when you have a bacterial infection.
- Call your doctor if you have frequent heartburn or poorly controlled nighttime asthma. Take the steps listed in this chapter to prevent heartburn.
- Contact your local YMCA, adult education center, hospital, or American Heart Association to find out about stress management classes in your area. Or, go to your local bookstore or library to get a book on stress management techniques so that you can learn them at home.
- Plan your next vacation according to locale, season, and your asthma triggers. See your health care

provider before you go and ask for a letter that describes your medical history, asthma management plan, and medications. Also, get the name of a doctor and hospital in the area where you'll be vacationing from either your doctor or a specialty organization, such as the American Academy of Allergy, Asthma and Immunology. Check Chapter 11, "For More Information," for a listing of additional resources.
- Prepare for you vacation by getting your medications refilled so you have enough to see you through your trip. Write a list of your medications—including the generic and brand name—along with the dosages and place the list in your wallet or purse.

Chapter 9

Living With Asthma: Through The Years

Throughout this book, you've learned that asthma isn't the same for everyone. By now, you know that the asthma symptoms you have might be different from those your friend has. Asthma varies between individuals. It also varies between different age groups. If you think about it, this age variation makes sense. An infant's lungs, for example, are less developed than an older child's. So an asthma attack could be more dangerous for a baby. For teenagers, the many details involved in managing asthma may threaten the teenager's emerging sense of independence. Therefore, their asthma management plans must be convenient. And older adults may be more sensitive to asthma medication. For them, choosing the right medicine in the right amount is critical.

This chapter explores the details of asthma for children and older adults. Here you will find information specific to these age groups, from triggers and medication to general questions of asthma management at home and school. As you read, you'll learn how asthma affects infants and preschoolers, children over 5 years old, and adolescents; ways to handle asthma treatment at school; and how asthma affects the elderly.

ASTHMA IN CHILDREN

Among kids, asthma is the most common chronic (lasting) illness. In the United States, over 4 million people under age 18—or more than one child in 20—have asthma. The wheezing, coughing, and complicated treatment can cause children to feel embarrassed, miss school, repeatedly visit the doctor, or even race to the emergency room. Very rarely, asthma that goes untreated for a long time may even lead to death.

And asthma is growing more common. Since 1980, asthma rates have more than doubled, and children are the most affected. Why is asthma such a problem for kids? We're still trying to find out—but we do have some ideas. For one thing, most children severely affected by asthma live in urban areas, where many asthma triggers, such as allergens, are prevalent. Cockroaches, which thrive in cities, also constitute a potent allergen difficult for children to avoid. In addition, most people are being diagnosed with asthma because we have better diagnostic tools. Finally, the trend toward tightly sealed homes, which allows indoor allergens (allergens from dust mites and cat or dog dander) to collect, is likely to be factors in the increase in asthma diagnoses.

Fortunately, asthma can be treated in kids, from the very young to teenagers. Today, a child with asthma doesn't have to miss out on soccer games or sit on the sidelines during recess. Kids of all ages can feel confident about their health. But they need their parents' help. As a parent, your job is to help your child learn how to control his or her asthma. That means avoiding asthma triggers, taking the right medication at the right time (and the right way), and monitoring breathing as needed. For younger children, you may need to do these things for the child. Let's start by looking at how asthma affects the youngest kids.

Children Under 5 Years Old

Up to three-fourths of children with asthma develop the condition in their first five years of life. Often, asthma begins as a viral respiratory infection. Instead of getting better quickly, a child's cough or labored breathing seems to linger. It's a good idea to see your child's health care provider when a cold seems to stick around. That's especially true for very young children, whose lungs are still developing and don't work as efficiently as those in older children.

Diagnosis

Diagnosing asthma in babies and young children can be tricky. The major problem is that wheezing, coughing, and hard breathing also can mean bronchitis, pneumonia—and more rarely, a variety of serious conditions, including cystic fibrosis (a rare genetic disease that causes lung problems), heart disease, and immune system disorders. To decide if your child truly has asthma, your doctor will do a detailed medical history and physical examination.

You can prepare for this visit by reading Chapter 2, "Working With Your Health Care Provider." If your child has anything beyond very mild asthma (characterized by just occasional symptoms), you should probably see an asthma specialist. If you are in a health maintenance organization (HMO), ask your primary care provider to refer you to a pediatric asthma specialist, usually an allergist.

Medication

Few studies have been done on asthma medicine in children under 3 years old. If your doctor thinks medication is needed, he or she might prescribe cromolyn, which has a strong safety record. It's likely that you'll try a short course of medication and see how your child's symptoms respond. Then, you might stop the medicine altogether. The kind and amount of medication will depend on the severity of your child's asthma. In general, doctors try to get asthma under control quickly and then slowly reduce the medicine level. This approach varies among doctors, however, and it may vary with the age of the patient.

Some drugs are not safe for infants. In particular, theophylline can be dangerous because it builds in the body during a fever, and fevers are common among babies. Ask your health care provider about asthma medication in infants.

Chapter 4, "Asthma Medications," explains the general varieties of asthma medicine and how they work. The most effective asthma medications are inhaled. These drugs go straight to the lungs, working quickly to relax the airways that spasm during an asthma attack and remain chronically swollen. Some young children can't use asthma inhalers, so they breathe in medication using a compressed-air machine called a nebulizer. This machine allows them to slowly inhale medication over the course of about 10 minutes. Usually, young kids wear a face mask to breathe in medicine; older children can use a nebulizer with a straw-like inhaler device. Nebulizers must be cleaned carefully and regularly so bacteria don't build up and get inhaled, causing infection. These devices also are discussed in Chapter 4.

When you have an infant with asthma, it's important to watch out for early symptoms of an asthma attack. With your health care provider, you will create an asthma management plan that lists, step by step, what to do when early symptoms appear (see Chapter 5, "Managing Your Asthma Day To Day"). Your management plan should include things like whether you go to the emergency room or doctor's office, how you'll get there, how much it will cost, who else you will notify, and who can watch your other children. Make copies of your management plan to share with family members, babysitters, or close friends. Also, keep a copy at work and home.

In general, you should go immediately to the emergency room if your baby's:

- skin starts looking pale or red
- chest starts to get big
- cry become shrill, short, and soft
- breathing rate increases
- suckling or feeding stops
- nostrils open wider
- skin between the ribs seems pulled tight

During an asthma attack, do not try to treat your baby at home by, for example, giving him or her lots of liquids. The key is to be prepared and get medical care quickly.

Children Over 5 Years Old

In some preschoolers, asthma symptoms gradually wane. Other kids end up with asthma throughout childhood. It's impossible to know which path your child might take. But according to the National Heart, Lung and Blood Institute, asthma that lingers throughout childhood often is associated with allergy, a family history of allergy or asthma, and exposure to passive smoke (usually cigarette) and asthma-causing allergens.

For school-age kids, asthma brings a special challenge. These children are learning how to get along with peers and work well in social settings, like school or extracurricular activities. It's important to nurture a child's self-esteem and control asthma at the same time. The solution is to take a team approach: together, you and your child will work with health care providers, teachers, school nurses, and coaches, as the case may be. Your job is to help your child understand how to control asthma and then provide the foundation with which to do it.

For these children, as for everyone with asthma, good health comes down to three things: avoiding asthma triggers, taking medication, and monitoring breathing. These topics are each discussed in previous chapters. You can learn about asthma triggers in Chapter 3, "Asthma-Proofing Your World." Depending on what triggers your child's asthma, you can take certain steps to help treat it. For example, don't smoke around your child. If you smoke, go outside to do it. You also may need to remove a pet or fluffy stuffed toys from your home, encase your child's bed mattress in plastic, or take other precautions.

Most children with asthma have what's called "allergic asthma," which is triggered by specific allergens. In the past, doctors frequently suggested immunotherapy, or allergy shots, for these children. Immunotherapy is not as commonly used today. New research suggests that asthma drugs usually can do the job by themselves.

When it comes to medication (discussed in Chapter 4), the trend is to treat a child's asthma aggressively, get it under control, and then slowly taper off medication to the lowest amount possible. The most common long-term controller medication for kids is cromolyn sodium (brand name: Intal®). The Food and Drug Administration also recently approved nedocromil sodium (Tilade®) for children 6 to 11 years of age. A variety of quick-reliever medications may be used.

Kids in this age group usually can use inhalers, but it's very important to teach them the right technique. Otherwise, they won't get the full benefit of their medication. It's also important to explain why taking asthma medicine on time is critical, even if your child feels fine. Several studies have shown that, if left to themselves, many kids forget to take the right amount of medication. We need to remind children to take their medicine in a positive way and praise them when they remember to do it on their own.

The last feature of asthma treatment, monitoring, is especially important in this age group. Chapters 2 and 5 offer tips for managing asthma. Regular check-ups at the doctor will help your child review inhaler technique, rethink asthma medication plans, and talk about any problems or questions. Encourage your child to talk with your doctor frankly. A few days before your visit, ask your child how he or she feels about the asthma management plan. Does the medication seem to work? Is your child still struggling with hard breathing or coughing? Do you have any questions for the doctor yourself? Maybe your child is considering going to camp, for example, or is worried that learning how to swim might be difficult because of asthma. Now is the time to ask.

At School

At home, your child probably can deal with asthma fairly easily. You two can talk about it openly, for example, or get medication as soon as it's needed. But life at school can be different. There are a lot of kids around, and a lot of things to do. Controlling asthma can get lost in the shuffle. What's more, every child wants to "fit in," and yours may feel embarrassed pulling out an inhaler or wheezing during gym class. That's why it's so important for you to help. Your child doesn't need to miss out on activities or feel uncomfortable because of asthma.

The best approach is to start dealing with your child's asthma before the school year begins—or right away, if school's already in session. Ask your doctor (and see organizations listed in Chapter 11, "For More Information") for books or articles explaining how asthma affects a school-aged child. Once you have this information, share it with your child's teacher and a school nurse. You might even put in a call to the school principal. These people need to know how asthma affects your child. For example, you'll want to consider things like:

- Triggers

    Classrooms sometimes contain asthma-causing allergens, like dusty carpeting or mold. If your child's asthma seems to get worse at school, these triggers could be to blame. Also, your child may need to be particularly careful during art or science projects that involve paints and other chemicals—strong odors can trigger asthma attacks in some people. The same thing goes for certain foods.

- Medication

    During an asthma attack, inhaling medication quickly is the fastest, safest route to relief. But schools have varying policies regarding medicine. Some schools don't let a child carry any drugs, even an asthma inhaler. When this is true, it's important that the school clinic keeps an inhaler with asthma medication for your child.

    Also, some kids will need to take medicine on a regular schedule. Make sure both your child and school personnel know when regular trips to the nurse's clinic are needed. It's essential that teachers and nurses help your child take medication without making a "big deal" out of it. That will help your child feel more confident.

    Some medicine may cause side effects, too. According to the American Academy of Allergy and Immunology, asthma medication might sometimes cause a child to have a headache, stomachache, shakiness (which might cause sloppy handwriting), sleepiness, or a hard time concentrating. If your child's ears get stuffy with nasal allergies, he or she might not hear as well.

Similarly, asthma can cause a cough or runny nose. These symptoms are not contagious, and a child does not need to be sent home. If any of the above things are true with your child, tell the teacher.
- Exercise

    One of the most common asthma triggers is exercise—especially intense exercise, like running, soccer, or basketball, which lead to heavy breathing. For most kids with asthma, there's no reason to sit on the sidelines. Exercise is important to everyone's health. So if your child has exercise-induced asthma, tell the coaches or physical education instructors. A teacher/coach needs to know what medication your child needs, how much medicine should be taken, when that medication should be taken, what to do if the medicine doesn't seem to help, and what to do during an emergency.

Usually, inhaling a puff or two of certain medications before exercise will allow your child to join in sports and games without problems (see Chapter 4). Sometimes, however, your child may need to adjust his or her activity. "Asthma and Physical Activity in the School," a report published by the National Heart, Lung and Blood Institute, offers these tips for helping your child enjoy exercise to the fullest. Share the advice with teachers/coaches:

- Include warm-up and cool-down times. Take this time to stretch and use medication as needed.
- Before beginning a new type of exercise, check a child's written asthma management plan, which should explain any limits on that child's activity.
- Also before beginning, check the environment for any known asthma triggers—for example, freshly cut grass or a newly-painted gym.
- Be alert to the symptoms (wheezing, labored breathing, coughing) of an oncoming asthma attack. If a child does have an attack, take care. Use medication as needed and let the child rest for a reasonable amount of time (possibly the remainder of the class or activity).
- Modify exercise according a child's ability. For example, rather than run a mile, an asthmatic child might walk part—or all—of the way.

If a child can't fully participate, be sure to involve him or her. Maybe a child with asthma can keep score, take care of equipment, or play a position that doesn't require a lot of running, like goalie. Suiting up and heading out on to the field with the other kids is important to every child's sense of self-esteem.

- Convenience

    Perhaps the biggest factor driving a student's success with asthma treatment is convenience. A child should be able to attend school even with mild symptoms. He or she also needs to get medication easily when needed. You, as a parent, need to be easy to reach if an asthma attack does occur. All these things boil down to preparation. Communicate with your child's school. If you provide written instructions for asthma care and easy access to medication, you're halfway there. Last, be sensitive to your child's self-esteem. The school-age years are full of peer pressure. Don't add asthma to it.

When To Stay Home

Sometimes it's hard to tell when your child should stay home or go to school despite asthma symptoms. If a child feels awful, of course, he or she should take the day off. But given a choice, many kids would do just this, no matter how they feel. That's why it's important for you to talk to your child and use a few specific measures to tell if today is a sick day.

In general, your child probably can go to school if he or she has just slight asthma symptoms, such as a little wheezing that responds to medicine, for example, or a runny nose without wheezing. A peak-flow meter can help you determine how well your child's lungs are working. If usual activities aren't a problem, then school shouldn't be, either.

On the other hand, there are times when kids with asthma definitely should stay home. If your child has any of the following symptoms, call the school. You might consider calling your doctor, too:

- A fever over 100 degrees

- Very fast or hard breathing
- Wheezing or coughing that lingers even an hour after taking medication
- An infection or the signs of one (sore throat or tender, swollen glands in the neck)
- A feeling of extreme weakness or fatigue
- A peak-flow reading at least 30 percent less than a personal best and that doesn't respond to asthma treatment

Adolescents

In terms of asthma symptoms and lung testing, adolescents tend to resemble children more than adults. The biggest difference about this age group is their need for independence. Teenagers may feel like asthma treatment is "a pain," or nuisance, and dismiss the condition.

The best solution is to actively involve a teen in his or her asthma management. This is not the time for you, as a parent, to make decisions for your child or relentlessly hammer home good health messages. In fact, many doctors find it helpful to visit with adolescents alone first, and then invite parents into the office. This gives the child a sense of respect and importance in asthma treatment. It also allows a health care provider to "connect" with young patients. Because some adolescents will hesitate to share their asthma stories with a doctor, questionnaires or other handouts may sometimes help.

In general, an adolescent—more than a parent—should help set goals for therapy, create a treatment plan, and review the effectiveness of that plan over time. As a parent, your job is to encourage your child and answer any questions that may come up. Working with adolescents can be like walking a fine line. You want to be supportive but not overwhelming. It's important to let your child make as many decisions as possible. The more in control he or she feels, the more likely asthma treatment will succeed. The National Jewish Medical and Research Center recommends that adolescents and their parents divide up health responsibilities this way:

An adolescent should:

- Create a written medicine plan
- Take medication and learn how to spot side effects
- Tell adults when a medication prescription needs a refill
- Learn how to take regular peak-flow readings, and keep up with it
- Discuss with an adult, on a regular basis, how asthma treatment is going

A parent should:

- Occasionally check medications and therapies
- Take on more responsibility during a child's stressful times or illness
- Routinely watch a child do peak-flow assessments to keep track of the readings
- Discuss with an adolescent, on a regular basis, how asthma treatment is going

OLDER ADULTS

For older adults, asthma brings a different set of challenges. As we age, a number of things tend to happen. First, we're more likely to come down with a variety of conditions and be taking medication for them. We're also more sensitive to most medications than younger adults. In addition, untreated chronic conditions, like asthma, can slowly get worse over the years, until some lung damage is irreversible.

All these things can complicate asthma diagnosis and treatment for older adults. For a long time, we didn't think of asthma as a problem for the elderly. But we've learned that asthma can occur at any time in life. Some adults will develop asthma after the age of 70, for example. Others may have the condition for years, but they aren't diagnosed until late in life. And diagnosis is the first step.

Diagnosis

In older adults, asthma can be difficult to diagnose because its symptoms are similar to common conditions, such as chronic obstructive pulmonary disease (COPD). This general term describes a number of lung conditions (particularly chronic bronchitis and emphysema) in which your lungs gradually become less efficient at inhaling and exhaling air. In other words, your lungs don't function as well as they once did. Heart disease also may cause asthma-like symptoms.

Elderly adults with asthma may cough often, feel a sensation of tightness in the chest, feel out of breath, and wake up at night frequently. To diagnose asthma, a health care provider will do a physical examination, take a medical history, and perform one or several specific lung function tests. (For more on diagnosis, see Chapter 2.) If a doctor is still uncertain, older adults might be asked to try an asthma medication. If symptoms respond, then asthma is probably the cause.

As for everyone with asthma, an asthma treatment plan involves avoiding asthma triggers, taking the right medication, and monitoring breathing.

Triggers

The common asthma triggers discussed in Chapter 3 affect young and old alike. But elderly adults seem to be particularly sensitive to asthma problems caused by respiratory infections and medication for other conditions. One solution is immunization. The National Heart, Lung and Blood Institute suggests that people between the ages of 60 and 75 get vaccinated against the pneumococcus bacterium every 5 to 7 years. Those over 75 should get vaccinated every 3 to 4 years. Also, an influenza vaccine is a good idea every year.

If you're an older adult with asthma, be sure to tell your doctor about any medicine you're taking for other conditions. If you have high blood pressure or coronary artery disease, for example, you may be taking a drug called a beta-adrenergic blocking agent ("beta blocker").

These drugs can aggravate your asthma. If you must take them, your doctor probably will recommend specific asthma drugs (ipratropium bromide) that will help with this side effect.

Other drugs that may aggravate your asthma or react with your medication include:

- some diuretics, or medication that promotes urination
- nonsteroidal anti-inflammatory drugs (NSAIDs), often used to treat arthritis
- some antibiotics and antihistamines, used to fight colds
- angiotensin-converting-enzyme (ACE) inhibitors, which help treat high blood pressure

Medication

To treat asthma, your doctor will recommend most of the same asthma drugs used by younger adults (and discussed in Chapter 4). However, your treatment plan depends on your response to medication and any other conditions you may have. For example, if you have COPD, you may use a bronchodilator more often than usual, and you may get less benefit from anti-inflammatory therapy. Ipratropium bromide may cause fewer tremors and heart palpitations than other asthma drugs. As always, the asthma therapy that works best depends on your own situation.

A few asthma drugs can cause complications in older adults. Theophylline may cause a fast heartbeat, nausea, insomnia, and liver disease. Oral (systemic) long-acting beta$_2$ agonists sometimes leads to tremors or too little oxygen in the blood. In older women, high doses of inhaled corticosteroids can worsen osteoporosis, a gradual weakening of the bones. This effect however, can be minimized by taking calcium and a vitamin D supplement. Estrogen may sometimes be added, too. Systemic corticosteroids can cause a range of problems, including high blood pressure, heart problems, and eye disease, and osteoporosis.

It's important that medications for older adults be convenient to use. If you have arthritis, for example, you may have a hard time using a hand-held inhaler to breathe in medication. A nebulizer could help. Or maybe you have difficulty keeping track of your medication. These are common problems, and you shouldn't hesitate to talk with your health care provider about them.

Management Plan

Every older adult with asthma benefits from regular check-ups—every three to six months—with a doctor. At these appointments, your health care provider will perform a peak-flow test to measure your breathing ability. Depending on the severity of your asthma, you also may do peak-flow readings at home. If peak-flow tests are too complicated or difficult to do at home, your asthma diary becomes important. (See Chapter 5 for more details.)

The idea, as in all asthma management, is to learn when your symptoms are growing worse and respond quickly. If you live with family members or you have in-home care givers, share your asthma treatment plan with them. They can help remind you to take medication or be on the lookout for worsening asthma symptoms. Last, of course, they can help during an asthma attack.

Despite differences in triggers, medication, and monitoring, all older adults with asthma should have one thing in common: comfort. You need to be comfortable with your asthma treatment plan. If you're not, then talk to your health care provider. Together, you can take steps to alter your approach. Some older adults feel confused or depressed about asthma. This shouldn't be the case. In fact, once you get your asthma under control, you'll feel much better than before. You'll breathe more easily and be more confident.

SUMMARY

- Asthma varies with age. Most children with asthma develop the condition before 5 years of age. These children are too young to understand an asthma

treatment plan. If your young child has asthma, you need to learn about the condition, remove asthma triggers from your home, and help your child take medication as needed. Your health care provider will help.
- For school-age kids, asthma can be a challenge. There's no reason for these children to miss out on school sports, stay home sick (often), or feel embarrassed about their asthma. Again you, as parent, play a critical role. You can inform your child's teachers, coaches, the school nurse, and others about your child's asthma. Make sure they have a copy of your family's asthma management plan—and make sure they understand how asthma affects your child in particular. This team approach can minimize asthma's impact and let your child stay active and involved.
- Adolescence—or the teen years—is a time of emerging independence. For these children, asthma can become a point of struggle with parents. Don't let it. Teenagers should take control of their asthma management plans. Let them decide what to do about triggers, how to take medication, and how monitoring will work. Be involved—but not overbearing—as a parent. This approach is the best way to keep a teen on top of his or her asthma.
- Asthma can be challenging for older adults, too. They may be more sensitive to asthma medication. They also may have existing conditions that mimic or aggravate asthma. For older adults, perhaps the most important feature of asthma management is comfort. Medication should be as convenient as possible, as should monitoring. Routine check-ups, every 3 to 6 months, can help ensure that an older adult is on the right track.

ACTION PLAN

This chapter is full of details that affect people of different ages. To better understand how these details fit into the broader picture, you might:
- Revisit chapters 3, 4, and 5. These chapters talk about

asthma triggers, medication, and monitoring. They can fill in basic information about asthma.
- Make notes or questions for your health care provider.
- Check out Chapter 11, "For More Information," to find support groups and information about asthma in children and older adults.

Chapter 10

Frequently Asked Questions

When it comes to asthma, there's a lot to learn. Having a few answers at your fingertips may help. Here are 20 frequently asked asthma questions. To learn more about each question, read the relevant chapter or contact the organizations listed in Chapter 11, "For More Information."

How do I know I have asthma? You can't tell you have asthma by judging your symptoms yourself. The wheezing, coughing, and breathing difficulty associated with asthma can also indicate other conditions, too. Your best bet is to see your doctor. Your health care provider will take your medical history, do one or several lung function tests, and perform a physical examination.

If I have asthma, does that mean my children will, too? Asthma does tend to run in families, so it's possible your children will develop the condition. But they may not. Researchers are still learning why some people develop asthma and others don't. If you have asthma, you should take steps to remove asthma triggers from your home. Removing triggers may help protect both you and your kids.

At the natural foods store, I found some herbal medicine with a label that says it can cure asthma. I've also read that antihistamines or general inhalers can help. Should I try these treatments? Most doctors and researchers advise against these over-the-counter (OTC) treatments for asthma. Asthma is a unique disorder in which your lungs don't work properly. The most effective medication acts in a precise way to help your lungs. These precise drugs are only available by prescription from your doctor. By contrast, OTC medication works in a general, hit-or-miss way. Depending on your asthma, OTC drugs may help a little—or not at all.

Do people die from asthma? When asthma is treated, its effects on the body are minimized. Most serious problems start when asthma is uncontrolled. For example, if you have asthma for years but you're not diagnosed, your lungs may gradually get worse. You're also more likely to get severe asthma attacks. Occasionally, asthma can lead to serious illness or even death. Some people die of asthma-related conditions more often than usual, including people with severe asthma or without medical care. African Americans—particularly those 15 to 44 years of age—are more likely to die from asthma than other ethnic groups.

How can I tell when an asthma attack is coming? That depends on your personal asthma symptoms. Usually, in the hours or days leading up to an asthma attack, your body sends signals that something is wrong. You may get an itchy or sore throat, feel short of breath, or begin coughing more than normal. Once you figure out what your personal warning signs are, you'll know when to expect an asthma attack. You can respond by checking in with your doctor, taking medication, and being extra careful to avoid asthma triggers.

What should I do during an asthma attack? The most important thing is to stay calm. With your doctor, you should create an action plan for what to do during an attack. Most people find inhaling a quick reliever medication can ease an asthma attack within 5 to 10 minutes. These drugs relax the airways in your lungs. Most asthma attacks last less than an hour. If you're having difficulty breathing, or if your symptoms do not improve after taking medication, call your doctor. If you're having a severe asthma attack that seems out of control, go to the emergency room immediately.

Is asthma the same thing as allergy? Not exactly. Asthma causes inflamed, or swollen, airways in your lungs.

Allergies are the most common "triggers," or causes, of asthma. However, some people only get asthma while doing exercise, for example. So you can have asthma without allergies and vice versa.

Is there a cure for asthma? No. But we can treat the condition better than ever before. With the right treatment plan, your asthma shouldn't slow you down.

I have a hard time talking to my doctor about asthma. What should I say? Be honest and clear with your health care provider. Before your appointment, make a list of all the questions and concerns you have. Chapter 2, "Working With Your Health Care Provider," can help. If you don't understand something, be sure to ask your doctor. Also, go over your treatment plan together. Don't be afraid to express concern. For your asthma plan to work, you must be comfortable with it. If you aren't, ask about making changes.

I want to get a pet. Are there any animals that won't make my asthma worse? There's no such thing as an "allergen-free" pet. Dogs, cats, birds, and rodents all carry allergens that can trigger asthma in sensitive people. If you are one of these people, your best bet is to not get a pet. If you already have one, ask your doctor how to keep your home as asthma-free as possible.

Are asthma medicines safe? No drug is completely free of side effects in everyone who takes it. But for the most part, asthma medication is safe. Inhaled medication, which works directly on your lungs, causes fewer side effects than oral (pill or liquid) medicine. Be sure to ask your health care provider about the safest medications (and amounts) if you're taking other medicine or have an existing medical condition. Also, certain medications are safer for kids and older adults.

I read about asthma studies in the newspaper all the time. Should I change my medication or try a new approach that's "in the news?" Before you make any changes to your asthma treatment plan, talk to your doctor. Asthma is different for different people, and what works in one study may not help your own condition. Together, you and your health care provider can decide to change your therapy.

If I'm taking asthma medication on schedule, why do I need to monitor my breathing at home? If you have moderate or severe asthma, monitoring your breathing with a peak flow meter can be important. Peak-flow readings tell you when your asthma is beginning to get worse—long before you can actually sense a change in symptoms. Similarly, consistently good peak-flow readings tell you that your asthma is under control and it might be time to scale back on medication.

If I have asthma, can I still exercise? Should I worry about having sex? Exercise is an important part of life. When it comes to relationships, so is sexual intercourse. You shouldn't give up either because of asthma. Don't be embarrassed to ask your doctor about these activities. Most of the time, inhaling asthma medication ahead of time can prevent wheezing or difficulty breathing.

Why does my asthma get worse in the spring? You may be allergic to outdoor pollens and mold spores that crop up this time of year. During the spring, tree and grass pollens can cause sneezing and wheezing. Your doctor can help you learn whether pollen is triggering your asthma. If so, you can take steps to avoid these triggers—by staying inside during times when the pollen load in the air is highest, for example.

I've just learned that I'm pregnant. Will my asthma make a difference? It could. During pregnancy, your asthma could worsen, improve, or stay the same. Some women develop asthma for the first time while pregnant. No matter what your situation, it's important to treat your asthma to ensure that your baby gets a steady supply of oxygen. Certain medications appear safe for pregnant women. You can also monitor your breathing and your baby's heartbeat. When treated, asthma does not usually affect pregnancies or child birth.

Can you outgrow asthma? The idea that you "outgrow" asthma is really more myth than reality. Many children do seem to have fewer asthma symptoms as they grow up. The condition may even fade into the background. But because asthma is a chronic disease, the possibility of an asthma attack never disappears completely. With your health care provider, you can monitor your health over the long term and decide what—if any—treatment you need.

I don't think my child's school is being helpful about her asthma. What can I do? First, make sure you have collected all the written information on asthma in school-age children. Your doctor may have pamphlets or brochures. Also, contact the organizations in Chapter 11 to ask them for information. Share the materials with your child's teacher, nurses, and coaches or physical education instructors. It's important that your child feels comfortable taking medication at school, eating lunch with the other kids, and participating in sports or activities. You can learn more about this in Chapter 9, "Living With Asthma: Through the Years."

Is asthma an emotional disorder? No. Because asthma varies so much from person to person, doctors once thought asthma was partly "in your head." But over the years, research has shown that asthma is a very real condition with certain triggers and lung reactions. It is not a psychological disorder. However, shouting, crying, or other emotional behavior may sometimes make an asthma episode worse.

If I follow my medication plan, avoid asthma triggers, and monitor my breathing, will I be able to control my asthma? Most likely, the answer is yes. It depends on the severity of your asthma. In general, when you have your asthma under control, you should experience few or no asthma attacks. Your breathing should be nearly normal. You shouldn't wake up at night coughing or wheezing. In short, you'll feel better and breathe better.

Chapter 11

For More Information

Here's a list of organizations that offer asthma information. Much of it is free. For example, you can learn about dealing with asthma at home or school, spotting asthma triggers, understanding medication, or even joining an asthma support group. The fastest route to information is often the Internet, so you'll find some Internet addresses on this list. You also can call these groups and request information by mail.

The websites listed below are useful sources of information, and there are countless sites on the Internet that feature asthma information. How do you separate the good from the bad? Here are some guidelines for finding credible asthma facts on the Internet—and anywhere else, for that matter:

* Be a skeptic. If it sounds too good to be true, then it probably is. Watch out for product promotions and biases, such as giving only the opinion of one person. Ask your doctor before making a change in your asthma management plan based on information you happen to come across.
* Know the source of the information. Trust information only from established organizations, such as hospitals, health associations, universities, and government agencies
* Look for an Internet site that shows when the information was last updated. You want a site that has been updated at least within the past month.

Allergy and Asthma Network/Mothers of Asthmatics, Inc.
3554 Chain Bridge Road, Suite 200
Fairfax, VA 22030-2709
1-800-878-4403
e-mail: aanma@aol.com
http://www.podi.com/health/aanma

American Academy of Allergy, Asthma and Immunology
611 Wells St.
Milwaukee, WI 53202
1-800-822-ASTHMA (1-800-822-2762)

American Academy of Pediatrics
141 North West Point Boulevard
Elk Grove Village, IL 60007
(847) 228-5008
http://www.aap.org

American College of Allergy, Asthma and Immunology
85 West Algonquin Road
Arlington Heights, IL 60005
1-800-842-7777
http://allergy.mcg.edu

American College of Chest Physicians
3300 Dundee Road
Northbrook, IL 60062
(847) 498-1400
1-800-343-ACCP
http:www.chestnet.org/

American Lung Association
For the affiliate nearest you and/or printed material, call 1-800-LUNG
USA: 1-800-586-4872
e-mail: ala@aol.com
http://www.lungusa.org
Offers information about local support groups.

American Thoracic Society
1740 Broadway
New York, NY 10019
(212) 315-8700
http://www.thoracic.org

Asthma and Allergy Foundation of America
1125 15th St. NW, Suite 502
Washington, DC 20005
1-800-7-ASTHMA (1-800-727-8462)

http://www.aafa.org
Offers information about local support groups.

Asthma Information Center
Journal of the American Medical Association
http://www.ama-assn.org/special/asthma
Healthfinder +
U.S. Public Health Service
http://www.healthfinder.gov

National Asthma Education and Prevention Program
National Heart, Lung and Blood Institute Information Center
P.O. Box 30105
Bethesda, MD 20854-0105
(301) 251-1222
http://www.nhlbi.nih.gov/nhlbi/nhlbi.htm

National Institute of Allergy and Infectious Diseases
National Institutes of Health
Building 31, Room 7A-50
31 Center Drive, MSC2520
Bethesda, MD 20892-2520
(301) 496-5717
1-800-243-7644
1-800-874-2572
http://www.niaid.nih.gov

National Jewish Medical and Research Center
1400 Jackson St.
Denver, CO 80206
1-800-423-8891
http://www.njc.org

National Technical Information Service
5285 Port Royal Road
Springfield, VA 22161
(703) 487-4650

Index

Page numbers in italics refer to figures.

Accolate (*see* Zafirlukast).
Acid reflux (*see* Heartburn, frequent).
Adolescents, 137
 management goals, 132–133
 parental responsibilities, 133
 special considerations, 132
Adults, older (*see* Older adults).
AeroBid, AeroBid-M (*see* Flunisolide).
Air, indoor (*see* Indoor air).
Air conditioning, 33
Air ducts, cleaning of, 34
Air-cleaning devices, 34
Albuterol, 39–40
Allergens
 animal
  questions regarding, 141
  ways to avoid, 27, 93
 cockroach, 27–28, 93, 124
 description of, 5–6
 food, 28–29
 house dust mites, 26–27, 93
 molds
  indoor, 28
  outdoor, 25–26
  tips for avoiding, 93
 outdoor pollens, 25–26
 types of, 22, *92*
Allergic rhinitis, 22–23
Allergies
 cause of, 23
 vs. asthma, comparison, 140–141

Allergist, 13–14
Allergy shots, 29–30, 94
Allergy skin testing, 29
Alupent (*see* Metaproterenol sulfate).
Amantadine, 112
Animal allergens
 questions regarding, 141
 ways to avoid, 27, 93
Anti-inflammatory drugs
 cromolyn sodium, 43–44, 97
 nedocromil sodium, 43–44, 97, 128
 nonsteroidal, 32
Appointment (*see also* Doctor).
 first, 15–17
 follow-up visits, 18–19
 preparations for, 14–15
 what to expect, 15–19
Asthma
 annual costs, 2
 causes of, 2
 control of, 143
 cough-variant, 83, 87
 day-to-day management (*see* Day-to-day management).
 exercise (*see* Exercise-induced asthma).
 frequently asked questions, 139–143
 incidence of, 2
 inheritance, 139
 levels of, 48–49
 management of (*see* Management plan).
 medical impact, 2
 mortality, 140

Asthma (*continued*)
  occupational (*see* Occupational asthma).
  organizations, 145–147
  seasonal, 83–84, 87, 142
  sexual activity and, 142
  treatment (*see* Medications).
  vs. allergy, comparison, 140–141
Asthma attacks
  in children under 5 years old, 126
  during pregnancy, 102–104
  how to deal with, 74–76, 140
  warning signs, 74–75, 140
Asthma diary
  how to use, 72–74
  illustration of, 73
  purpose of, 71
  sample entries, 72
Attacks, asthma (*see* Asthma attacks).
Azmacort (*see* Triamcinolone acetonide).

Baby, unborn, asthma effects on (*see* Pregnancy).
Beclomethasone dipropionate (Beclovent), 42–43, 96
Beta$_2$ agonists
  long-acting, 44–45, 97, 135
  short-acting, 39–40, 95
Bitolterol mesylate, 39–40
Breast feeding, medication use and, 98
Breathing, monitoring of during pregnancy
  asthma attacks, 103–104
  considerations for, 98–100
  questions regarding, 142
Brethaire (*see* Terbutaline sulfate).
Bronchodilators (*see* Quick relievers).

Childbirth, 102–103
Children, asthma in
  under 5 years old
    diagnosis of, 125
    medications, 125–126
    onset of, 124
    summary, 136–137
    symptoms that warrant emergency attention, 126
  over 5 years old
    allergens, 127
    considerations at school
      exercise, 130
      medication, 129–130
      overview, 128–129
      triggers, 129
    management approach, 127
    medications, 127–128
    monitoring, 128
    when they should stay at home, 131–132
  prevalence of, 123–124
  social effects, 123–124
  triggers, 124
Chronic obstructive pulmonary disease, 134
Cigarette smoke (*see* Tobacco smoke).
Cockroach allergen, 27–28, 93, 124
Common cold
  choice of medication, 111
  description of, 119–120

INDEX

management of, 110
prevention, 111–112
symptoms of, 110
COPD (*see* Chronic obstructive pulmonary disease).
Corticosteroids (*see also specific medication*).
   during pregnancy, 96
   how to take, 42
   inhaled types, 42
   oral types, 42
   osteoporosis and, 135
   when to take, 42
Cough-variant asthma, 83, 87
Cromolyn sodium, 43–44, 97

Dander, 85
Day-to-day management
   action plan, 78
   asthma attacks, 74–76
   asthma diary, 71–74
   color-based management plan, 69–71
   overview, 65–66
   peak-flow meters
      how to use, 68
      personal best, 68–69
      when to use, 68
      who should use, 65
Decadron Phosphate Respihaler (*see* Dexamethasone sodium phosphate).
Dehumidifiers, 34
Delivery of baby, 102–103
Deltasone (*see* Prednisone).
Devices, for administering medications
   inhalers (*see* Inhalers).
   nebulizers (*see* Nebulizers).
Dexamethasone sodium phosphate, 42–43

Diary, asthma
   how to use, 72–74
   illustration of, 73
   purpose of, 71
   sample entries, 72
Doctor (*see also* Appointment).
   action plan, 20
   how to find the right one, 12–13
   how to talk with, 12, 141
   preparations to see, 14–15
   questions to ask, 13
   role in management plan (*see* Management plan).
Dry powder inhaler (DPI), 56
Dust mites (*see* House dust mites).

Elderly (*see* Older adults).
Exercise
   considerations for school-age children, 130–131
   effect on triggering of asthma, 32
Exercise-induced asthma
   description of, 79–80
   diagnosis, 80–81
   management plan, 81–83
   medicine plan, 81
   sports activities, 82
   summary of, 87
   trigger, 80

Fetal monitoring, 103
Flu
   management of, 112
   prevention, 113
   vaccine, 113
   virus types, 112

Flunisolide, 42–43
Follow-up visits, 18–19
Food allergens, 28–29
Fragrances, 31
Frequently asked questions, 139–143

Gastroesophageal reflux disease (GERD)
  bronchospasms and, 115
  description of, 114, 120
  management of, 115
  prevention, 115

Hay fever, 22–23
Health care provider (*see* Doctor).
Heartburn, frequent, 114–115, 120
HEPA filters, 33–34
Histamine, 23
House dust mites, 26–27, 93
Humidifiers, 33

Illness, symptoms of, 109–110
Immunizations, for older adults, 134
Immunotherapy, 29–30, 94
Indoor air, devices that affect
  air conditioning, 33
  air ducts, 34
  dehumidifiers, 34
  description of, 32–33
  humidifiers and evaporative coolers, 33
  indoor air-cleaning devices, 34
  vacuum cleaners, 33
Indoor molds, 28
Influenza (*see* Flu).

Inhaled medications
  advantages, 126
  beta$_2$ agonists (*see* Beta$_2$ agonists).
  corticosteroids, 42
  during pregnancy, 94–96
  inhalers (*see* Inhalers).
  learning to use, 52–53
  vs. oral medications, 52
Inhalers
  for children
    under 5 years old, 126
    over 5 years old, 128
  considerations when using, 59
  dry powder, 56
  metered dose (*see* Metered dose inhaler).
  nebulizers (*see* Nebulizers).
  new advances in, 55–56
Intal (*see* Cromolyn sodium).
Intensive fetal monitoring, 102
Ipratropium bromide, 135
Irritants (*see also* Allergens).
  description of, 22, 92
  strong odors and sprays, 31
  tobacco smoke, 30
  wood smoke, 31
  in workplace, 85
Isocyanate, 84

Labor, asthma considerations during, 102–103
Leukotriene antagonists, 3, 45–46
Liquid Pred (*see* Prednisone).
Long-term medications
  administration using inhalers (*see* Inhaled medications).

INDEX   **153**

corticosteroids (*see* Corticosteroids).
cromolyn sodium, 43–44, 97
during pregnancy, 96–97
guidelines for use, 46
how they work, 41
leukotriene antagonists, 3, 45–46
long-acting beta$_2$ agonists, 44–45
nedocromil sodium, 43–44, 97

Management plan
asthma attacks, 75–76
color scheme for, 69–71
day-to-day (*see* Day-to-day management).
for exercise-induced asthma, 81–83
goals of, 17–18
green, yellow, and red colors, 69–71
medications (*see* Medicine plan).
for occupational-induced asthma, 86–87
personal best peak-flow number, 68–69
for pregnancy
avoid triggers, 92–94
medications, 94–98
monitoring, 98–103
step-down vs. step-up approach, 49–50
ways to tailor, 17–18
Material Data Safety Sheets, 85
Maxair (*see* Pirbuterol acetate).
MDI (*see* Metered dose inhaler).
Medical history, 15–16

Medications
benefits of, 37–38
breast feeding and, 98
for children
under 5 years old, 125–126
over 5 years old, 127–128
considerations for using, 47–48
during pregnancy, 94–98
effect on triggering of asthma, 32
forms, 6
long-term
administration using inhalers (*see* Inhaled medications).
corticosteroids (*see* Corticosteroids).
cromolyn sodium, 43–44, 97
during pregnancy, 96–97
guidelines for use, 46
how they work, 41
leukotriene antagonists, 3, 45–46
long-acting beta$_2$ agonists, 44–45
nedocromil sodium, 43–44, 97
management of, 59–60
over-the-counter, 38, 98, 139–140
quick-relief
administration using inhalers (*see* Inhaled medications).
during pregnancy, 95–96
guidelines for using, 41
short-acting beta$_2$ agonists, 39–40
theophylline, 40–41

Medications (*continued*)
  safety of, 141
  types of, 6
  what to expect, 37–38
Medicine plan
  evaluation of, 60–61
  management of, 59–60
  medications (*see* Medications).
  for mild asthma, 48
  for moderate asthma, 48
  for severe asthma, 49
  step-down and step-up approaches, 49–50
  tips for, 50–51
Medrol (*see* Prednisolone).
Metaproterenol sulfate, 39–40
Metered dose inhaler
  cleaning, 55
  common mistakes when using, 54
  description of, 52
  how to determine amount of remaining medicine, 55
  how to use, 53–54
  spacers, 54–55
Metocorten (*see* Prednisone).
Metrapel (*see* Metaproterenol sulfate).
Mild asthma
  description of, 48, 67, 90
  treatment plan for, 48, 67
Mites (*see* House dust mites).
Moderate asthma
  description of, 48, 67, 90
  treatment plan for, 48, 67
Molds
  indoor, 28
  outdoor, 25–26
  tips for avoiding, 25–26, 93

Nebulizers
  for children under 5 years old, 126
  cleaning
    daily, 57–58
    every two weeks, 58–59
  how to use, 56–57
Nedocromil sodium, 43–44, 97, 128
Nonsteroidal anti-inflammatory drugs, 32

Occupational asthma
  diagnosis of, 85–86
  incidence of, 84
  management plan, 86–87
  summary of, 87–88
  triggers, 84–85
Odors, strong, 31
Older adults, 137
  considerations for, 133
  diagnosis, 134
  management plan, 136
  triggers, 134–135
Oral corticosteroids
  during pregnancy, 96
  how to take, 42
  side effects, 43
  types of, 42
Orasone (*see* Prednisone).
Organizations, 145–147
Outdoor molds, 25–26
Over-the-counter medications, 38, 98, 139–140

Panasol (*see* Prednisone).
PDE4 inhibitors (*see* Phosphodiesterase inhibitors).
Peak expiratory flow rate, 66, 99–100, 102–103
Peak-flow meters
  for children, 131

cleaning, 68
description of, 16, 66, 99
for determining triggers, 69
function of, 66
how to use, 68
personal best, 68–69
use during pregnancy, 99
when to use, 68
who should use, 66–67
Pediapred (*see* Prednisolone).
PEFR (*see* Peak expiratory flow rate).
Pets (*see* Animal allergens).
Phosphodiesterase inhibitors, 47–48
Physical examination, 16
Physician (*see* Doctor).
Pirbuterol acetate, 39–40
Pollens, 25–26
Prednisolone, 42–43
Prednisone (Prednicen-M), 42–43, 96–97
Preeclampsia, 90
Pregnancy, asthma during
  action plan for, 106–107
  asthma attacks, 102–104
  breast feeding considerations when taking medications, 98
  breathing, monitoring of, 98–100
  diagnosis, 99
  how it affects you, 90–91, 142
  how it affects your baby, 8, 91
  labor and delivery considerations, 102–103
  management plan
    avoid triggers, 92–94
    medications, 94–98
    monitoring, 98–103
  medications
    long-term controllers, 96–97
    quick relievers, 95–96
    rules for taking, 94–95
    unsafe types, 97–98
  monitoring considerations
    for you
      during first trimester, 99–100
      during second trimester, 101
      during third trimester, 101–102
    for your baby
      during first trimester, 100
      during second trimester, 101
      during third trimester, 102
  preeclampsia, 90
Pregnancy (*continued*)
  special conditions that warrant attention
    anxiety, 105
    diabetes, 105
    rhinitis, 22–23, 105
    sinusitis, 105
  treatment goals, 91–92
  triggers, 92–94
Presurgical considerations, 115–116, 120
Proventil (*see* Albuterol).

Quick relievers
  administration using inhalers (*see* Inhaled medications).
  during pregnancy, 95–96
  guidelines for using, 41
  short-acting beta$_2$ agonists, 39–40
  theophylline, 40–41

Respbid (*see* Theophylline).

Salmeterol, 44–45
School-age children, asthma in, 137
  allergens, 127
  considerations at school
    exercise, 130
    medication, 129–130
    overview, 128–129
    questions regarding, 143
    triggers, 129
  management approach, 127
  medications, 127–128
  monitoring, 128
  when they should stay at home, 131–132
Seasonal asthma, 83–84, 87, 142
Senior citizens (see Older adults).
Serevent (see Salmeterol).
Severe asthma
  description of, 49, 67, 90
  during pregnancy, 102
  nebulizer use (see Nebulizers).
  treatment plan, 49, 67
Sexual activity, 142
Sinusitis
  description of, 113
  management of, 113–114
  prevention, 114
  symptoms of, 113
Slo-Bid (see Theophylline).
Slo-Phyllin (see Theophylline).
Smoking (see Tobacco smoke).
Sonogram, 100
Spacers, 54–55
Specialists, asthma, 13–14
Spirometer, 16
Sports, for people with exercise-induced asthma, 82
Sprays, 31
Sterapred (see Prednisone).
Stress, and asthma
  management strategies, 117
  relationship between, 116–117, 120
Sulfites, 28
Surgery, preparations for, 115–116, 120

Teenagers (see Adolescents).
Terbutaline sulfate, 39–40
Tests, medical, 17
Theophylline (Theo-24, Theo-Dur, Theolair)
  for children under 5 years old, 125
  during pregnancy, 96
  how to take, 40
  for older adults, 135
  side effects, 40–41
  when to take, 40
Tilade (see Nedocromil sodium).
Tobacco smoke, 31, 93
Tornalate (see Bitolterol mesylate).
Traveling
  tips for, 118–120
  triggers, 118
Treatment plan (see Management plan).
Triamcinolone acetonide, 42–43
Triggers
  definition of, 21
  exercise, 32
  exercise-induced asthma, 80
  inhalant allergens (see Allergens).

irritants
  description of, 22
  strong odors and sprays, 31
  tobacco smoke, 30
  wood smoke, 31
  in workplace, 85
medications, 32
occupational irritants, 32
occupational-induced asthma, 84–85
in older adults, 134–135
peak-flow meters to determine, 69
questions to determine, 23–25
types of, 5, 22
weather, 31

"Twitchy lungs," 2

Uniphyl (*see* Theophylline).

Vacuum cleaners, 33
Vanceril (*see* Beclomethasone dipropionate).
Ventolin (*see* Albuterol).

Weather, as trigger of asthma, 31
Wood smoke, 32
Workplace-related asthma (*see* Occupational asthma).

Zafirlukast, 45–46
Zileuton (Zyflo), 45–46

WITHDRAWN

JOHNSON CITY PUBLIC LIBRARY
JOHNSON CITY, TN

12/12/1998

WITHDRAWN